The
Bird Flu
Pandemic

The
Bird Flu
Pandemic

CAN IT HAPPEN?
WILL IT HAPPEN?

How to Protect Yourself and
Your Family If It Does

Dr. Jeffrey Greene

with Karen Moline

THOMAS DUNNE BOOKS | ST. MARTIN'S GRIFFIN ≉ *New York*

THOMAS DUNNE BOOKS.
An imprint of St. Martin's Press.

www.stmartins.com

ISBN 0-312-36056-8
EAN 978-0-312-36056-6

First Edition: March 2006

10   9   8   7   6   5   4   3   2   1

A NOTE TO READERS

This book is dedicated to the millions who perished in the Spanish Flu pandemic of 1918–1919. May the knowledge of their sacrifices help protect future generations from the scourge of bird flu pandemics.

CONTENTS

The
Bird Flu
Pandemic

INTRODUCTION

I had a little bird/Its name was Enza/I opened up the
window/and in-flew-enza.
—*Popular children's rhyme in 1918*

It started with a cough, or perhaps a sore throat and a nose that needed blowing. It often ended a day or two later—sometimes, shockingly, within hours—with patients literally drowning in their own blood, their bodies suffocated into a blue hue so pronounced that exhausted nurses placed morgue-ID tags on their toes before they'd drawn their last breath.

What killed these patients so swiftly and so terribly?

Influenza.

That influenza, nicknamed the Spanish Flu, although it was certainly not Spanish in origin, was not a sweet little bird. It was an incomprehensible, raging, terrifying monster. Isolated cases of what was thought at first to be seasonal flu early in 1918 suddenly morphed into a pandemic that in one month alone—October 1918—nearly 200,000 Americans perished. Around the world, entire communities were destroyed. No one will ever be able to tell how many died, but the current estimate is between 80 and 100 million souls.

If the 100 million figure is accurate, that means that one-sixteenth of the world's population at that time had been killed by the flu.

Then, as swiftly as it arrived and spread, the Spanish Flu disappeared.

The pandemic was so horrible that it effectively reduced life expectancy in our country by thirteen years, yet it was so painful to remember that it was literally erased from our history books.

It took decades for scientists to realize that a virus was responsible for the pandemic. Only very recently have scientists been able to reconstruct the actual genetic structure of that particular strain of virus, and be unpleasantly surprised at what they discovered.

The lethal 1918 influenza was caused by a bird virus.

Somehow, a virus that had infected one species had managed to mutate into something that could infect another species. Namely, *us.* Human bodies had never been exposed to such a virus before. There was no natural immunity to it. As soon as the bird flu shifted from a few instances of *birds* infecting people . . . to *people* infecting people, the stage was perfectly set for a global pandemic.

Which brings us to this book. Back on May 21, 1997, in Hong Kong, a small boy died from a very specific strain of the flu. At that time, several hundred people became ill, eighteen were hospitalized, and six of them died.

The strain that killed them was the bird flu, called H5N1.

Since then, a wary—and as yet still incomplete—global watch has been set up to track the possibility of bird flu once again mutating from *birds* infecting people . . . to *people* infecting people. If this H5N1 virus suddenly becomes transmissible from person to person, it could turn into a global pandemic in the time it takes a jumbo jet to wing its way around the world.

Can such a pandemic happen again?

Yes. In addition to the 1918 pandemic, there were two other influenza pandemics in the twentieth century (in 1957 and 1968). The bad news about those pandemics is that bird viruses contributed to both.

Is another pandemic happening now?

No.

Or rather—*not yet.*

When will it happen again?

That's the $800 billion question. That sum being the bare-minimum figure the World Bank has bandied about in terms of economic losses should an influenza pandemic arrive.

Why is everyone so worried now?

Because the H5N1 avian influenza is most definitely on the move.

"Something has happened to the relationship between the virus and wild birds that hadn't happened before," said epidemiologist Michael Osterholm, director of the U.S. Center for Infectious Disease Research and Policy.

Ever since chickens started dying in Asia in 2003, this outbreak has become the most severe ever seen. Over 100 million chickens have died or been culled in thirteen different countries. No longer confined to poultry, the virus is appearing in ducks and other migratory birds who've flown on their usual flight paths from Asia through Russia to Europe, or from Asia over Alaska and into Canada and America.

Let's not forget that America is the world's largest producer and exporter of poultry meat and the second-largest egg producer—an industry valued at $23.3 billion in 2003. What if our chickens start to get sick?

The H5N1 virus that has killed so much poultry in Asia has also killed people in Vietnam, Cambodia, Indonesia, Thailand, and China, who've had close contact with chickens and roosters. As of early January 2006, 142 people have been become clinically ill with avian influenza, and 74 have died. The mortality rate for those who've been infected hovers close to the 50 percent mark, which is not a good sign. (Seasonal flu kills about 36,000 people in the United States, with a mortality rate of less than 0.25 percent. The 1918 pandemic had a mortality rate of about 5–12 percent; the exact figure can never be known, as the exact death toll was impossible to calculate.)

Worse, there have been several cases where it has likely been transmitted person-to-person. That is *definitely* not a good sign.

Right now, H5N1 is still predominantly a danger to poultry and birds. It has *not* yet been reported in America. Of course it could be here and we just don't know it yet.

Which means we must be vigilant. H5N1 has infected people. It has killed people. This is what sets the stage for a possible pandemic. The real tipping point will happen when there are clusters of human cases that could only be explained by person-to-person transmission.

This will happen only if and when H5N1 undergoes a significant mutation.

Is that happening now?

We just don't know.

Can it happen soon?

It *might*. If it does happen soon, I'd say we're in real trouble. If we have some time, we might not be.

The possibility of a pandemic hasn't stopped the media from conflating H5N1's possible leap from birds to people into the end of the world as we know it. Naturally, creating terrifying worst-case scenarios sells lots of newspapers and greatly improves ratings on TV, so a certain amount of sensationalism is always going to accompany any stories about what could be a very dire situation.

The operative word when it comes to the current bird flu situation, of course, is *could*.

Some of the near-daily reports in the media and on reputable government websites are clear, calm, and based on solid science and carefully evaluated risk factors. Some of them aren't. The result, as with any scare, is a lot of hype and hysteria. I can attest to that because my office phone is ringing off the hook. I have over 4,000 patients, and many of them are terrified, their fears fueled by the hype-mongers out there. What is Tamiflu™? they ask. Can I get it, right this minute? How do I use it? How do I know if I have the bird flu? Why is this happening?

It's so important to stress the unpredictability of where we are right now. I'm reminded of those analysts on Wall Street who state with absolute clarity and conviction that the markets are going to respond one way or the other; they're not right any more than they're wrong.

Same thing with the bird flu. Odds are extremely high that there will be a viral pandemic at some point in the foreseeable future. (There have always been viral epidemics and pandemics, and always will be—if that's any consolation! As I'll discuss in chapter 1, the difference between pandemics and epidemics is largely one of magnitude.) Will it be caused by H5N1? If not, what will be the causative virus, and where will it strike first?

What is known is that in the worst-case scenario, a flu pandemic would have a catastrophic impact on every aspect of our lives. A 50 percent mortality rate would kill half those infected—an unimaginable figure. With a clinical attack rate of 5 percent, we could anticipate 6,250,000 deaths and an equal number of seriously ill persons in our country alone. The economic impact would be in the hundreds of billions.

But I don't think we should get carried away just yet. Be realistic, certainly—but realize, too, that there are many differences between the 1918 pandemic and the possibility of another one.

On a positive note:
- We know what viruses are, how they cause influenza, and can track their mutations.
- We understand the H5N1 virus better now than we did when it first appeared. We know which host species are involved. We have learned that the elimination of sick birds reduces the possibility of transmission. The fewer people exposed to the virus, the less likely it is to have the chance to mutate into something more lethal.
- We can be stunned by the announcement in mid-November 2005, that China was beginning an audaciously ambitious plan to vaccinate all its birds against the H5N1 strain. There are 14 *billion* birds in China!
- We have anti-viral drugs, and vaccines to prevent some viruses.
- We have technological know-how.
- We have antibiotics to treat the secondary bacterial infections that often killed flu victims after the virus had run its course.
- Hospitals have pandemic emergency plans in place.
- Hygiene and sanitation are vastly improved.
- We have government-supervised surveillance of disease outbreaks, called the National Biosurveillance Initiative in America, to help, according to the U.S. Department of Agriculture, "rapidly detect, quantify and respond to outbreaks of disease in humans and animals, and deliver information quickly to state and local and national and international public health officials."
- Even the White House has made the possibility of a bird flu pandemic a central focus of its domestic policy. President Bush outlined a $7.1 billion strategy in early November 2005, to prepare for the danger of a pandemic influenza outbreak, saying he wanted to

stockpile enough vaccine to protect 20 million Americans against the current strain of bird flu. (As of December 2005, Congress had approved only 3.8 billion.)
- Most of the other countries around the world are aware of the seriousness of the situation.
- We have the Internet and means of transmitting information globally within seconds.

But, in other ways, we're not so far away from 1918 as we might hope.

On a negative note:
- There is no magic bullet cure for influenza. Nor will there ever be. Viruses mutate. They mutate quickly. They will *always* be able to mutate.
- Vaccines often take years to develop, require accurate predictions as to the precise strains likely to cause outbreaks, and may not be effective in every person vaccinated.
- Many more Americans lived on farms and in small towns in 1918. Once a primarily rural country, America now has most of its citizens living in large cities. The larger the population living in close quarters, the larger the probability of their getting infected.
- The ease of international travel makes the spread of a virus extremely easy. In 1918, it took about six weeks for the Spanish Flu to infect the world. Now, it could take less than six hours. Plus, we weren't worried about sick flocks of Chinese chickens back then.
- We know that some migratory birds can carry this strain and not get sick, which means they're more likely to spread the virus than birds that keel over and die on farms.
- China's audaciously ambitious plan to vaccinate all its 14 billion birds may be a logistical impossibility.
- People are still misinformed and Internet hypesters ("Buy this mask now! Kill bird flu virus!") certainly don't help.
- Despite many improvements, our government is still woefully unprepared for a sudden global catastrophe.
- Hospitals may have emergency plans in place, but they likely will be overwhelmed by the sheer numbers of the infected who will be seek-

ing treatment. They lack the necessary surge capacity for large numbers of critically ill persons.

• Other countries, lacking in funds and expertise, will be unable to establish any kind of vigilant surveillance prior to a pandemic, or any kind of thorough treatment during a pandemic.

• Many people are connected to the Internet and have the ability to transmit information globally within seconds. Yes, it's a great way to inform people of emergency instructions during a pandemic or other crisis—to stay at home and away from crowds, for example. But it may also cause many to rush to an already-infected and overcrowded hospital where they'd be exposed to far more danger.

• People are still likely to panic in the worst-case scenario.

Although the previous anthrax and SARS virus scares thankfully did not translate into mass casualties, explaining precisely what these diseases are—allaying fears and remaining calm—is a challenge. Most people have a hard time understanding selective mutation, evolutionary biology, and the science behind vaccine and drug development, and I can't say I blame them. Disease *is* hard to understand.

Plus, from my perspective as an infectious disease specialist, I can tell you that most people's expectations are simple—but dangerously misguided. The expectations are that we can control infectious diseases, and that people don't die prematurely of infectious diseases.

That just isn't true. It never will be true.

One thing we do know for certain is that flu viruses are sneaky and unpredictable. They evolve. They mutate. They shift from benign to lethal and back again.

That doesn't mean that H5N1 is going to be the virus that kills millions.

This book will be a comprehensive guide to everything you need to know about bird flu (and about all flu and previous pandemics). Part of my job is explaining complicated medical information to patients who don't have an advanced knowledge of science—but need to understand what I'm telling them so they can understand their illness and be compliant with their treatments. Most of the chapters are written in a question/answer format, so you can quickly turn to specific sections and read what's there without getting bogged down in incomprehensible data.

It is my hope that this book will become essential reading for all who are concerned about the flu, need to know what to do should the worst happen, and want to be proactive about every aspect of their health.

No one can stop a virus from mutating. But we can stop the panic, the hysteria, the hoarding, and the hype—and help everyone understand what they can do to keep themselves safe.

We can also take heart. The catastrophic pandemic of 1918 didn't kill off planet Earth. We're still here. Whenever the next pandemic arrives, some if not most of us will survive it, too. Instead of worrying, I hope everyone can seize upon our current situation as a wake-up call for preparedness in the case of a future flu pandemic, or a natural disaster, or a biological terror attack. The Boy Scouts have their sensible motto for a reason: Be Prepared.

Part I

A BRIEF HISTORY
of PANDEMICS

Chapter 1.

A BRIEF HISTORY *of* FLU PANDEMICS

The epidemic is seldom mentioned, and most Americans have apparently forgotten it. This is not surprising. The human mind always tries to expunge the untolerable from memory, just as it tries to conceal it while current.

—*Critic H. L. Mencken, writing about the*
1918 Spanish Flu pandemic

Isn't it interesting how "pandemic" and "panic" share the first three letters?

For as long as there has been recorded history, there have been pandemics. For those unlucky enough to fall victim to them, the operative word is often "panic." It's hard not to panic when death strikes down people in their prime, seemingly at whim and with cunning precision.

In the uneasy balance between all living creatures and the diseases that plague (literally!) them, sometimes the diseases are going to lash out—and win. During the thirteenth century, the bubonic plague pandemic, caused by the *Yersinia pestis* bacteria and transmitted by the bites of tiny rat fleas, killed an estimated 300 million people.

Eight centuries later, despite the astonishing advances and complete transformation of society and science, we're still at war with disease. And the sad, irrefutable truth is we always will be. Viruses and bacteria appeared billions of years before we did. They're not going anywhere in a hurry.

Yet there's a huge difference between the plague years of the thirteenth century and the current years of HIV, SARS, anthrax, Ebola, and the newest virus, H5N1. In the early Middle Ages, no one had a clue what caused these devastating diseases to break out, kill, then disappear. Now, we have a vast knowledge of what makes these infectious agents such deadly foes—which means we can fight back.

Before we can fight, of course, we must know our enemy.

WHAT IS A PANDEMIC?

As earthquakes, volcanic eruptions, tsunamis, and floods wreak havoc on the world, so do pandemics. It can be stated with unerring precision that natural and biological disasters *will* occur each century. We still can't say with anything close to unerring precision *when* these disasters will occur. We can only be prepared for them.

As I mentioned in the Introduction, a pandemic is defined by *Merriam-Webster's Dictionary* as "occurring over a wide geographic area and affecting an exceptionally high proportion of the population." An epidemic is defined as "affecting or tending to affect many individuals within a population, community, or region at the same time." The difference is in size and scope.

President Bush got it right in a speech about the bird flu on November 1, 2005. "A pandemic is unlike other natural disasters," he explained. "Outbreaks can happen simultaneously in hundreds, or even thousands, of locations at the same time. And unlike storms or floods which strike in an instant and then recede, a pandemic can continue spreading destruction in repeated ways that can last for a year or more."

Pandemics disrupt every aspect of life, to put it mildly. They overwhelm the medical system, as few of the millions seeking treatment are able to find a hospital bed. Fear and quarantines keep people from work and children from school. Public meetings are shunned, or banned outright. Society as we know is put on temporary hold until the most lethal wave starts to ebb.

As the ability to travel long distances over trade routes became more established when civilizations developed, so grew the ability of viruses and bacteria to tag along for the ride. Historians of ancient Greece wrote about pandemics. They were also written about in detail in 1510, 1580, 1688, 1699, 1847–48, and 1889–90.

In the twentieth century, there were three pandemics of Type A influenza viruses: the Spanish Flu of 1918–1919, the Asian Flu of 1957, and the Hong Kong Flu of 1968.

The Spanish Flu pandemic was an H1N1 virus, and one of the greatest calamities of history, killing an estimated 80 to 100 million people in a little over a year. I'll discuss it at length starting on page 16.

Viruses that had mutated in *birds* caused all three of the pandemics of the twentieth century. These viruses then became communicable from birds to people, and then from person to person. Each virus was unique, however. What caused such a huge discrepancy in the total death toll from these pandemics was not how contagious these viruses were, but how much disease they caused. The sicker that people become, and the more quickly that they become very sick, the easier it becomes for them to die.

Usually, the flu kills the very young and the very old, but the 1918 Spanish Flu was extremely unusual in that it caused so much disease in young, healthy adults, aged 15–40. They succumbed by the millions, often only a day or two after first becoming ill. The disease in them was incredibly virulent. It often spared their children and their parents and took them instead.

Somewhere in the world, someone is getting sick with the plain old miserable flu right now. Although this plain old miserable group of viruses kills an average of 36,000 people in this country each year, many more people are sickened and then recover after a few days or weeks. Even with those kinds of fatalities, "ordinary" flu is not considered an epidemic-sized problem. For an influenza pandemic to take off, many different elements must come together and then occur simultaneously. That's not very easy to do, which is why pandemics, thankfully, happen infrequently. (The concept is not dissimilar to those combinations of forces that allow the formation of hurricanes: the prevailing upper wind currents must be moving just so; the temperature of the ocean must be warm enough; and other pressure systems must steer clear, for example.)

The stage is set for pandemics when four conditions have been met:

1. A virus pathogenic for humans establishes a global presence in an animal reservoir
2. There must be a new flu virus subtype to which the population is immunologically naïve (in other words, have no immunity)
3. The new virus infects people, and they get seriously ill
4. The virus is easily spread from person to person

Therefore, pandemics begin when a specific virus becomes easily transmissible from person to person, on a global scale. The virus doesn't just strike people in, say, California, or perhaps South Africa. It hits thousands of different locations *at the same time.*

It becomes uncontainable.

Not only must this virus be easy to transmit, but it must be one against which people don't have any immunity. This is the *sine qua non* of flu pandemics. Without this lack of immunity, a pandemic absolutely cannot happen.

Unfortunately, H5N1 has now fulfilled three of the four steps.

1. A virus pathogenic for humans establishes a global presence in an animal reservoir
2. It is a new virus in people (although it's not a new virus in birds)
3. It has infected 142 people, with a 50 percent mortality rate. The early cases in Vietnam had a 70 percent mortality rate.

If H5N1 mutates into an easily transmissible virus any time soon, no one on this planet will have any natural immunity to it.

But, H5N1 has *not yet* shown any propensity to make that crucial jump.

Even if an H5N1 pandemic started soon, we would not be able to predict the attack rate (how many get infected), or the mortality rate (how many die) until people started to die. The Spanish Flu had an attack rate of between 33 to 50 percent; at its height, *half the world* was infected. Although that figure is fairly unimaginable, equally disturbing is the mortality rate in the United States, which was 2.5 percent.

PANDEMIC STAGES

The World Health Organization (WHO) has divided the development of a pandemic into six stages. Right now, the H5N1 virus has caused a Stage 3 alert. Still, it is not yet anywhere close to either epidemic or pandemic levels.

Pandemics tend to come in waves. During the first wave of the 1918 Spanish Flu, the virus was extremely contagious and slightly more lethal than the usual seasonal influenza, but not an overwhelming killer. The second wave was devastating. It developed and then peaked within a period of two months. The third wave started several months later. Final waves of pandemics usually begin within a year of the initial outbreak.

Stage 1
Inter-pandemic phase — Low risk of human cases

Stage 2
New virus in animals, no human cases — Higher risk of human cases

Stage 3
Pandemic alert — No or very limited human-to-human transmission

Stage 4
New virus causes human cases — Evidence of increased human-to-human transmission

Stage 5
New virus causes human cases — Evidence of significant human-to-human transmission

Stage 6
Pandemic — Efficient and sustained human-to-human transmission

THE HORROR OF THE SPANISH FLU 1918–1919

The year was 1918, and King Alphonse III of Spain had the flu.

Unlike its neighbors, Spain was not at war. There were no censors monitoring its newspapers, so reporters there breathlessly followed their king's condition with concern, especially as millions of other Spaniards were falling like dominoes with a particularly nasty bout of the flu.

The king recovered. Many of those infected by the flu sweeping through Europe did not. Just how bad this flu truly was would not be reported in the newspapers of Spain's neighbors, where strict censors deleted anything that could remotely affect the morale of their soldiers mired in miserable fighting.

All these reports in Spain gave the flu its name—although in Spain, they called it the French Flu.

And this flu was certainly not Spanish in origin.

It was *avian* in origin.

The Spanish Flu originated in birds, then somehow mutated into a virus that could kill like no other disease since the Black Plague of the thirteenth century.

The first wave

Historians of the Spanish Flu have not been able to come to a consensus about its Ground Zero, and they may never be able to. Most think it started in the American Midwest. Virologist John Oxford is convinced that a precursor was somehow spawned in an English war camp in Etaples, France, in 1916. Then it was called purulent bronchitis, and it killed quickly, with a distinctive feature. As they approached death, those infected turned a distinctive shade of deep blue, called heliotrope cyanosis. Their bodies, desperate to breathe, literally raided the blood vessels in the face for oxygen.

As quickly as the outbreak began, it ended.

The camp at Etaples was an ideal breeding ground for flu outbreaks. Over two million British soldiers were stationed there at some point, and they were constantly on the move. (In the twelve hospitals were 20,000 beds, mostly to treat the wounded and shell-shocked.) The men were tired, anxious, and stressed, to put it mildly, and they weren't exactly living in the lap of hygienic luxury. There were farms on the camp with pigs and poultry to feed the hungry soldiers. Scavenging wild birds hovered nearby. And foreign nationals from most of the countries in the British Empire worked in the camp, breathing the same air and being exposed to the same germs before returning home to their own countries when the war ended.

Wherever the Spanish Flu pandemic actually originated, the first wave appeared in Haskell County, Kansas, in March 1918, in Camp Funston, an encampment that was part of the sprawling Fort Riley. Over 26,000 soldiers were training there, waiting to be shipped off to the harbor of Brest in France to fight in the Great War.

First the camp's cook became sick early on March 11. He said he had a "bad cold." By noon, over 100 other soldiers were sick as well. A week later, 500 were sick. Forty-eight of them died from what was listed as pneumonia.

For nearly 10 percent of otherwise strapping young soldiers who'd suddenly taken ill to die of what they first thought of as a "bad cold" was unheard-of. Strapping young soldiers did not die in army camps from colds—or from the flu, for that matter.

Many other soldiers took to their beds that cold spring. Some got sick in transit to other camps. Others fell ill while crossing the Atlantic. Over 84,000 "doughboys" shipped off in March; 118,000 followed in April. Some were bound to catch colds and the flu from each other, right? Still, one regiment of the Fifteenth U.S. Cavalry suffered thirty cases of the flu. Six quickly died. One in five! This was terrible news.

But if the news about this virulent flu spread, the soldiers might not be able to sail. Their training might be truncated. The balance of the war might shift.

So the Americans kept sailing.

Once the doughboys landed in Brest, they coughed on the French soldiers, who coughed on the Belgians, the English, the Germans, and anyone else they encountered. Within a month, all of Europe had outbreaks of the flu. It reached Bombay, then Shanghai by the end of May. There were 31,000 cases in the UK in June, with hundreds dying.

Although this flu was more lethal than usual—and, most worrisome,

it seemed to fell healthy young adults with brutal rapidity—those who
recovered tended to be better after only a few days. The outbreaks were
dubbed "Three-Day Flu" in Europe. And as cases seemed to wind down
as summer approached, those fighting the war got back to the business of
death and destruction. They thought the worst was over.

It wasn't.

The second, killer wave

World War I didn't just kill the estimated 15 million souls who perished
between 1914 and 1918. It created the ideal situation for a flu virus to
thrive. For that reason, the Spanish Flu and the war will always be inex-
tricably intertwined.

With the Spanish Flu, the close proximity of farm and wild birds to
an incredible concentration of weary soldiers from a worldwide demographic (who under normal circumstances would never have been in
such tight quarters in several countries) gave the virus a vast new supply
of hosts in which to percolate and take its time before making that final
mutation to lethality. Then, somehow, it made the jump from birds to
people. Combine that with the continuous movement of the troops
meant the virus could easily be spread all over the world in a much
shorter time than usual. This is why, in retrospect, it's not a surprise that
a pandemic would start toward the end of a war, when millions of people
who otherwise would not have been in a relatively small area were able to
disperse.

The troops brought it home with them.

By the end of August, many American soldiers were coming home on
leave, and they often disembarked at Commonwealth Pier in Boston
Harbor.

On August 28, 1918, there were eight cases of the flu in these returning soldiers. A week later, there were 119, most of whom were transferred
to the Naval Hospital in Chelsea.

From there, the flu spread to Camp Devens, which was thirty miles
west of Boston and temporary home to over 45,000 soldiers, crammed
into uncomfortable and unsanitary barracks.

The acting surgeon general of the army, colonel and former president of the American Medical Association, Victor Vaughn, was swiftly summoned to the camp by mid-September, and he was shocked to hear that sixty-three soldiers had died that very day. Throughout Massachusetts, over 50,000 soldiers and civilians were sick.

"I saw hundreds of young stalwart men in uniform coming into the wards of the hospital," he said. "Every bed was full, yet others crowded in. The faces wore a bluish cast; a cough brought up the bloodstained sputum. In the morning, the dead bodies are stacked about the morgue like cordwood."

One of the most eminent pathologists of his day, Dr. William Henry Welch, had also been summoned to Camp Devens. Perplexed and deeply worried about the mortality rate, he got to work. When he opened up the chest of a newly dead soldier, he was flabbergasted to see lungs that were engorged with blood. The normally soft and spongy lung tissue had become hard and thick, looking more like liver than lung.

"This must be some new kind of infection," Dr. Welch muttered. "Or plague."

It wasn't a plague. It was the Spanish Flu.

In the months between what would turn out to be a much more mild pandemic during the Spanish Flu's first wave, the virus had mutated. It was no longer the three-day flu. It was a relentless killer.

The seasonal strains of influenza are respiratory viruses that first destroy the epithelial cells of the upper respiratory tract. These cells are designed to protect the lower reaches of the bronchial tree and the lungs. If they are destroyed, it is possible to get sick with influenza (viral) pneumonia, as well. This explains why the very young and the very old, as well as the immuno-compromised, are most likely to die from the flu each year.

Not healthy young adults. Not soldiers in the peak of health.

Like all other flu, this new strain had a rapid onset. Patients developed a cough and a high fever. They often had headaches, and muscle aches, and a profound lassitude. Unlike seasonal flu, however, the Spanish Flu killed with astonishing speed. It upended the normal get-sick-feel-crummy-get-better scenario. It was able to burrow so deep inside the lungs, so early in the illness, that they became flooded before any immune

A LETTER FROM THE PANDEMIC FRONT LINES

This letter was written by a recently recruited military physician, Dr. Roy Grist, assigned to Camp Devens, a Massachusetts army base. It was found in a trunk in 1959, among other papers given to the Department of Epidemiology at the University of Michigan, and first published in the December 22, 1979, issue of the *British Medical Journal.*

Camp Devens, Mass.
Surgical Ward No. 16
29 September 1918

My dear Burt,

   Camp Devens is near Boston, and has about 50,000 men, or did have before this epidemic broke loose. It also has the base hospital for the Division of the Northeast. This epidemic started about four weeks ago, and has developed so rapidly that the camp is demoralized and all ordinary work is held up till it has passed. All assemblages of soldiers taboo. These men start with what appears to be an attack of la grippe or influenza, and when brought to the hospital they very rapidly develop the most viscous type of pneumonia that has ever been seen. Two hours after admission they have the mahogany spots over the cheek bones, and a few hours later you can begin to see the cyanosis extending from their ears and spreading all over the face, until it is hard to distinguish the colored men from the white. It is only a matter of a few hours then until death comes, and it is simply a struggle for air until they suffocate. It is horrible. One can stand it to see one, two or twenty men die, but to see these poor devils dropping like flies sort of gets on your nerves. We have been averaging about 100 deaths per day, and still keeping it up. There is no doubt in my mind that there is a new mixed infection here, but what I don't know. My total time is taken up hunting rales, rales dry or moist, sibilant or crepitant or any other of the hundred things that one may find in the chest, they all mean but one thing here—pneumonia—and that means in about all cases death.

   The normal number of doctors here is about 25 and that has been increased to over 250, all of whom (of course excepting me) have temporary orders— "Return to your proper station on completion of work"—Mine says, "Permanent Duty," but I have been in the Army just long enough to learn that it doesn't always mean what it says. So I don't know what will happen to me at the end of this. We have lost an outrageous number of nurses and doctors, and the little town of Ayer is a sight. It takes special trains to carry away the dead. For several days there were no coffins and the bodies piled up something fierce, we used to go down to the morgue (which is just back of my ward) and look at the boys laid out in long rows. It beats any sight they ever had in France after a battle. An extra long barracks has been vacated for the use of the morgue, and it would make any man sit up and take notice to walk down the long lines of dead soldiers all dressed up and laid out in double rows. We have no relief here; you get up in the morning at 5:30 and work steady till about 9:30 p.m., sleep, then go at it again. Some of the men of course have been here all the time, and they are *tired*.

If this letter seems somewhat disconnected overlook it, for I have been called away from it a dozen times, the last time just now by the Officer of the Day, who came in to tell me that they have not as yet found at any of the autopsies any case beyond the red hepatitis stage. It kills them before it gets that far.

Good-by old Pal,

"God be with you till we meet again"

Keep the Bouells [bowels] open,

Roy

response, however feeble, was possible. Bodies, starved for the oxygen that could not get into the super-inflamed lungs, developed the distinctive heliotrope cyanosis. Patients drowned in their own blood and fluids.

Worse, the progression from feeling fine to being near death from this extremely virulent type of pneumonia often took less than twenty-four hours.

In addition, many with the flu also suffered from epistaxis, or severe nosebleeds. Others bled from every orifice. Some women hemorrhaged so heavily from their vaginas that doctors initially thought they were miscarrying. This was the ultimate, cruel irony, for the Spanish Flu turned out to be the most lethal of all in pregnant women, killing them as well as their unborn children.

As the losses in the military barracks continued to mount, the flu continued its assault, moving west and engulfing entire towns in its wake.

No one knew what was causing this devastating illness, but many doctors and scientists became convinced it was due to a bacteria, Pfeiffer's bacillus, and they threw considerable energy into creating a vaccine.

It was a logical assumption, however, for at the time, viruses were unknown. (They wouldn't be identified for another fifteen years.) They are so infinitesimal that they can only be viewed with an electron microscope, which was decades away from being developed. And as viruses aren't living creatures like bacteria, no vaccine and no antibiotic could do anything to stop them in their tracks. (For more, see chapter 2.)

In nearby Boston, thousands were seriously ill. Plus they had no idea if they had the flu caused by a bacteria (bad enough) or were being poisoned (thoroughly terrifying). Rumors were flying that German spies had deliberately seeded Boston Harbor with influenza-sprouting germs, no thanks to Lt. Col. Philip Doane, head of the Health and Sanitation Section of the Emergency Fleet Corporation. On September 17, he publicly declared that "It would be quite easy for one of these German agents to turn loose influenza germs in a theater or some other place where large numbers of persons are assembled. The Germans have started epidemics in Europe, and there is no reason why they should be particularly gentle with America."

Two weeks later, 202 Bostonians died on a single day, October 2—not from German germ warfare, but from viral warfare. All public meeting places were ordered closed.

The corrupt city fathers and their cronies in Philadelphia did not ban assemblies as those in Boston had done. Dr. Wilmer Krusen, director of the Philadelphia Department of Public Health and Charities, was a political appointee who didn't know much at all about public health. He dithered, choosing to fall for the pabulum spooned out by Surgeon General Rupert Blue of the United States Public Health Service. Surgeon General Blue sent press releases to the newspapers, with information about how to treat the flu. "Bed rest, good food, salts of quinine, and aspirin for the sick," he declared.

Public health officials all over the country told people to stay calm. Royal Copeland, health commissioner of New York City, announced, "The city is in no danger of an epidemic. No need for our people to worry."

He had to eat his words. On one particularly awful day not long after, 851 people died in New York City from the flu (October 23).

In Los Angeles, the public health director announced, "If ordinary precautions are observed there is no cause for alarm." Forty hours later, public gatherings at schools, churches, and theaters were banned.

The procrastination of these officials proved to be disastrous—and especially so in Philadelphia. The fourth annual Liberty Loan Drive to raise money for war bonds had been scheduled for September 28. Even though over 200 people had been admitted to local hospitals the day before, desperately ill with the flu, Krusen decided to go ahead with the rally, as he'd been told in no uncertain terms that the city needed to fulfill its quota of war bond donations. The parade had been months in the planning. The country was at war, after all, and residents were intensely patriotic. They needed a day of fun to lift their spirits.

So the joyful spectacle wound its way through streets jammed with spectators. Over 200,000 people attended.

In a little over a week, most of them had the flu. Philadelphia was dying.

Everything was ordered shut.

"Don't get frightened or panic-stricken over exaggerated reports," Krusen said, but by then it was too late.

During the first week of October, there were 2,600 dead. On the worst day in Philadelphia's history, October 10, 1918, 759 perished.

During the second week 4,597 died, solely due to flu—a mortality rate 700 times higher than normal.

In one month, there were 11,000 fatalities in Philadelphia alone.

Doctors and nurses who could still stand in the overflowing hospital wards were so overwhelmed that bodies lay piled in heaps in the city morgue. The stench and filth was indescribable, and the doors lay open. No morgue workers went near the bodies; they were too fearful for their lives. Anyone could walk in to see them.

Not that anybody would.

The warm days of a beautiful Indian summer belied the horror enfolding in homes throughout the city. No one came to pick up the dead bodies, and they began to pile up on porches. Eventually, priests and seminarians became the only ones who could stomach the pick-up of so many dead bodies, wrapped in makeshift shrouds, before loading them haphazardly onto trucks and wagons. Families had to dig the graves of their loved ones themselves. There was not a coffin to be had or a gravedigger to be found.

"Don't Get Scared," read the headlines in the newspapers.

In his masterful and brilliantly detailed chronicle of the pandemic, *The Great Influenza,* author John M. Barry quoted many eyewitnesses to the horror.

"The fear in the hearts of people just withered them. They were afraid to go out, afraid to do anything," said Philadelphia hospital volunteer Susanna Turner. "You just lived from day to day, did what you had to do and not think about the future. If you asked a neighbor for help, they wouldn't do so because they weren't taking any chances.

"Even if there was war, the war was removed from us, you know—on the other side," she added. "This malignancy . . . it was right at our very doors."

A Washington, D.C., resident, William Sardo, was equally blunt: "It took away all your community life, you had no school life, you had no church life, you had nothing," he said. "People were afraid to kiss one another, to eat with one another, to have anything that made contact because that's how you got the flu. It destroyed these contacts and destroyed the intimacy amongst people. You were constantly afraid because you saw so much death around you, you were surrounded by death. When each day dawned you didn't know whether you would be there when the sun set that day. It wiped out entire families from the time that the day began in the morning to bedtime at night—entire families were gone completely, there wasn't a single soul left and that didn't happen just intermittently, it happened all the way across the neighborhoods. It was a terrifying experience."

People in cities stayed indoors, away from their neighbors. Handshakes were banned. Face masks became mandatory, although they were made from flimsy gauze and offered little protection from the virus. Rural Americans often had no idea of the extent of the national devastation. Many relied on folk remedies—garlands of onions and garlic, poultices of goose grease—that were as ineffective as they were noxious.

October 1918 became the deadliest month in this nation's history.

In thirty-one awful days, the flu would kill nearly 200,000 Americans. The Spanish Flu pandemic did not only terrify and kill Americans—

it circled the globe, indiscriminately striking those in its path. In Europe, 70,000 American soldiers got the flu. Some of the units were almost entirely stricken. In total, over 40,000 American soldiers died.

Other countries suffered staggering losses as the pandemic progressed. Some people literally collapsed and died, as if struck by lightning—the only mercy being that they didn't suffer. On one grotesquely memorable, three-mile-long streetcar ride in Cape Town, South Africa, the conductor, driver, and five other people died from the time the route started until its bitter end.

But a miraculous thing began to happen. As mysteriously as it had first appeared, the flu seemed to disappear. On October 26, the ban on public gatherings in Philadelphia was lifted. By November 11, people again flocked to the streets to celebrate the Armistice ending the Great War.

For many, though, it was too soon to celebrate.

The third wave

The Spanish Flu was dying down in America, or so it seemed. On November 21, residents of San Francisco were given the go-ahead to shred their face masks. Soon thereafter, however, there were 5,000 new cases of the flu.

Thankfully, the third wave was not as deadly to Americans as the second. Many who'd gotten sick in the first wave seemed immune to the second; those who survived the second didn't catch the third. The virus was mutating. But it continued to kill, just the same.

By April 1919, it was gone for good. H1N1 finally ran out of hosts to infect.

Historians estimate, on the conservative side, that at least 675,000 Americans died in all three waves of the pandemic, with most of the deaths between mid-September and early December. This figure is higher than the body count of all Americans who died in combat in all the wars of twentieth century.

At one point, *over half the 1.6 billion people* in the world in 1918 were infected.

Entire villages in Africa, Asia, and Central America were decimated.

Only those lucky enough to live where there were strict quarantines,

RECREATING THE 1918 FLU VIRUS

Astonishingly, the virus didn't disappear completely from the world.

Pathologists desperate to discover what was causing the Spanish Flu risked their lives to perform autopsies on newly deceased bodies. Samples from some of this lung tissue were preserved in formalin, placed on slides, carefully labeled, then forgotten, buried for decades with millions of other samples in the archives of the Armed Forces Institute of Pathology (AFIP), where researcher and pathologist Dr. Jeffrey Taubenberger is the chief of the Molecular Pathology Division. He was thrilled to find the slides containing tissue from two soldiers (one from Fort Jackson, South Carolina, the second from Camp Upton, New York), which he reported in 1997. Then, pathologist Dr. Johan Hultin was able to dig up the frozen remains of a Native Alaskan woman in Brevig Mission, Alaska—where nearly everyone had died from the flu in November 1918—and, amazingly, her lung tissue also retained viral material that could be extracted and studied.

Obviously, seeing how and why this virus was so lethal is critical to helping us understand how and why H5N1 is behaving as it is.

Using a technique called polymerase chain reaction, Taubenberger and his colleagues were able to extract and sequence the genetic material from the virus, and make stable, non-lethal copies of it to study and manipulate. They could also compare the virus to current strains to search for similarities and vital changes.

When Taubenberger's team recreated the H (the hemagglutinin protein) sequence of the H1N1 virus, they discovered a crucial shift compared to other bird flu strains. In 1918, the H had been slightly altered so that it could enter and bind to its human host cells with exceptional tenacity. In addition, they saw that H1N1 shows a fairly high degree of homology, or similarity of the gene's base pairs between the avian and the human strains.

What was the most surprising to the researchers was that the H1N1 virus was totally avian in origin. It hadn't made the jump from bird to another host animal (such as a pig) and then to humans, as hybrid viruses commonly do. It had jumped straight from birds into people, where its tenacious efficiency allowed it to spread so quickly.

Once the H1N1 viral sequence was complete, scientists were able to use it to recreate the actual, deadly virus itself. Using the highest level of precautions, a team at the Centers for Disease Control and Prevention (CDC) was able to inject a minute quantity into mice to follow its progression, which they reported in both *Nature* and *Science* magazines.

The infected mice got very, very sick: 39,000 times more virus particles were released from their lung cells four days day after infection than were released with the more typical, seasonal flu virus. All the mice died within six days of infection.

With subsequent tests, researchers found that newly infected mice responded to anti-viral medications. That was extremely heartening news.

"By identifying the characteristics that made the 1918 influenza virus so harmful, we have information that will help us develop new vaccines and treatments," Dr. Terrence Tumpey, the senior microbiologist at the CDC who recreated the virus, said. "Influenza viruses are constantly evolving, and that means our science needs to evolve if we want to protect as many people as possible from pandemic influenza."

such as in Australia, escaped the brunt of the flu's contagiousness. On November 7, 1918, for example, a ship from Auckland, New Zealand, docked in Western Samoa. Two months later, a staggering 22 percent of the islanders were dead. Those in American Samoa, about one hundred miles away, imposed such a strict quarantine that they had no contact with the outside world for months. No one there died.

For many years, the global death toll stood at 20 million, but that figure is now seen as improbably low. It's estimated that 20 million died in India alone. As it's impossible to ever tally an accurate reckoning, especially in large countries like India, China, and Russia, the current thinking is that approximately 80 to 100 million people perished worldwide. That would have been about one-sixteenth of the world's population at the time.

What was most devastating about this pandemic was how it attacked healthy adults. Some believe that up to 10 percent of young adults in the world died. According to Barry, the highest death toll was in adults aged twenty-five to twenty-nine, the second greatest was thirty to thirty-four, and the third twenty to twenty-four. Few people over the age of fifty died.

Why did people in their twenties die so easily? Scientists still aren't sure, but they think that the robust immune system of a healthy adult was somehow over-triggered by the virus. If that's true, it wasn't the flu virus alone that was so lethal—it was the body's overwhelming effort to rid itself of the invader that flooded their lungs, turned them blue, and ended their lives.

It is also thought that those over fifty had already been exposed to a variant of the H1N1 virus decades before, which may have given them partial immunity.

The Spanish Flu killed much more than its victims. Millions of children were orphaned, their lives and families shattered forever. Many of those who survived were left with brain damage. In his book, *Awakenings,* Dr. Oliver Sachs wrote memorably about the millions who developed encephalitis lethargica, a devastating condition in which victims were trapped in a twilight world of permanent sleep.

Some historians believe that the course of the world was altered as well, when President Woodrow Wilson got a nasty bout of the flu during the third wave. In France at the time, negotiating with the French victor, Georges Clemenceau, and the German generals, a weakened and less perspicacious Wilson made concessions to the forceful Clemenceau that many now think set the stage for World War II.

With a terribly sad poignancy, the Spanish Flu pandemic was all but erased from the history books until quite recently. I think that because the global death toll was severely underestimated, and historians were preoccupied with the devastation caused by World War II, this pandemic seemed (unfairly) insignificant in comparison. Plus, there's a certain protectiveness in modern medicine that makes such global devastation almost inconceivable to us now. And it's only human nature to want to forget things that are too horrendous to contemplate.

OTHER FLU PANDEMICS OF THE TWENTIETH CENTURY

While understandably devastating for anyone who lost loved ones, we were fortunate that the subsequent two pandemics of the twentieth century were far less lethal than the Spanish Flu.

Still, both originated in birds. They were caused by an antigen shift, where genes from a bird flu virus mixed, melded, and recombined with a human flu virus, and spawned two brand-new strains, H2N2 and H3N2.

1957–1958: Asian Flu

The H2N2 strain appeared in China at some point in early 1956, originating from a flu virus mutation in wild ducks combining with a pre-existing human strain. It spread to Singapore in February 1957, and to Hong Kong in April. It reached America in June.

Due to increased surveillance and scientific know-how, the race began to produce a vaccine. It was first available in America in August. Still, many school-age children got sick as the school year began, and spread the flu to their friends and families.

The flu seemed to be contained by the end of 1956, but a second wave suddenly started up, this time killing mostly the elderly in January and February of 1958.

This was typical flu virus behavior, as it were. Due to small viral mutations, a flu strain can first seem to go after certain demographic subsets of the population, calm down if not disappear entirely, then reappear to strike another segment of the population.

The total death toll was approximately 69,800 in the United States, and about one million worldwide. It could have been much, much worse.

1968: Hong Kong Flu

Also originating in wild ducks, the H3N2 strain first appeared in Hong Kong early in 1968. By September there were some cases in the United States; the largest amount of deaths took place during the peak months of December 1968 to January 1969 (also the peak death season for the annual flu). Unlike the Asian Flu of 1957–58, this strain was initially most lethal to the elderly.

Fewer people died during this pandemic, as the shifts in the virus only occurred in the H, not the N, so anyone who'd been alive during the 1957–1958 pandemic might have developed partial immunity to it. (I'll explain this in the next chapter.)

The total death toll was 33,800 in the United States, and at least 700,000 worldwide (estimates vary). It was thankfully the mildest pandemic of the past century.

2006: H5N1?

Once Dr. Taubenberger was able to genetically sequence the 1918 virus, we discovered that it looks very, very similar to H5N1. And since the structure of a virus dictates its function, virulence, and pathogenicity, we might be in for trouble.

H5N1 might mutate into a virus that will cause a devastating global pandemic. But then again, it might not. Much of what causes viral mutations and spread is still a mystery. We still don't know *how* the Spanish Flu managed to jump from birds to people and then from person to person.

As I'll discuss in subsequent chapters, unlike desperate physicians and scientists in 1918, we do have the means to fight back, with vaccines, anti-viral medications, and antibiotics to treat the opportunistic secondary infections that cause so much death in those already weakened by the flu. The Spanish Flu was so virulent that it killed many of its victims incredibly quickly with viral pneumonia; they literally didn't have a chance to get socked with a debilitating or lethal bacterial pneumonia.

This is the first time in history that we've literally been able to study a new virus as it mutates, compare notes, and come to a consensus on how to respond. In addition, global surveillance gives us a foothold in countries where the virus is spreading in birds, in the hopes that the World Health Organization and local governments can oversee its containment.

Epidemiologists do agree on one point: If H5N1 is not the virus that causes a pandemic, someday, somehow, somewhere, another one will.

Part II

ABOUT *the* BIRD FLU

Chapter 2.

THE ABCs *of* INFLUENZA VIRUSES, *or* ALL ABOUT *the* FLU

In order to understand what the bird flu is and why it's such a threat, we need to go back to the basics about viruses, seasonal influenza, and bacteria.

We'll never know exactly where viruses initially came from, as there will never be such a thing as virus fossils to study or accurately date. Suffice to say that viruses have been around for billions of years. Primordial life as we know it is presumed to have begun with a soup of chemicals all those billions of years ago, that somehow coalesced into life forms capable of using chemical substances as energy sources. Starting in the sea and then moving onto land, these earliest life forms developed the ability to use organic molecules for a variety of metabolic functions. These included the ability to form cellular structural integrity, the ability to resist the dangers of the environment, the capability of replicating, and the means to produce a sustainable source of energy from which the other cell functions could draw.

From the primitive cellular organisms that evolved in the earliest chapters of the Earth's history, came more and more complex multicellular organisms. Humans, most would argue, are the latest and most complex version of cell-based evolutionary process. Our genetic material

(DNA) shares elements with many other forms of life that coexist with us today, and are testaments to the commonality of our origins.

The viruses that have most likely shared our planet for several billion years have also evolved, but in a very different manner than the cellular organisms we know as living things. Rather than using evolution to develop the metabolic functionality shared by all living things, viruses have evolved in their ability to invade a wide array of life forms.

ALL ABOUT VIRUSES

What is a virus?

A virus is a geometrically shaped hollow structure that is so minute that thousands—or millions, depending on its size—can fit on the head of a pin. The geometry of the outer shell of the virus is dictated by its chemical composition and the shape of the protein components. (A useful comparison is a snowflake; each possesses a distinct shape that is determined by the infinite ways water molecules can assemble themselves.) The shell, or outer coat of the virus, is inert, but it is critical to the persistence and infectivity of the germ.

This is because the shell's molecular structure is perfectly adapted to invade specific hosts . . . and once it does, it can then evade the hosts' immune system, target specific cells within that host, bind to the target cell, enter the cell, and then inject its genome (contained within the viral structure) into that cell.

It is inaccurate to think of viruses as small living organisms. In fact, viruses cannot use the environment to produce energy; they cannot persist for extended periods on their own in the world; and most important, they are incapable of reproducing or propagating themselves on their own. Therefore, viruses are actually not living entities. I like to think of viruses as minute Pandora's boxes that must be delivered to a cell before they can be opened.

What viruses are especially good at doing is invading a living organism (the host) and using the host's cells to perform the functions that it requires to replicate. Viruses have been identified to use almost every form of living organism as hosts, from primitive bacteria and one-celled amoeba, to plant life, and all forms of higher animal life, including of course, mankind.

For this reason, it's not hyperbole to refer to viruses as the ultimate parasites. They are totally dependent upon a host for their persistence on the planet.

An apt comparison is to think of the host cell as a busy office where many activities are concurrently taking place. The "office" has copy machines. When the virus enters the cell, it is capable of directing the copy department to drop its jobs-in-progress, and to begin copying the viral genome (DNA or RNA) instead. Once the viral genome has been copied, the cellular "office staff" then reads those copies to assemble viral proteins according to the specifications of the viral DNA or RNA code.

As a result, each different virus targets a specific host for the purpose of co-opting its cellular machinery so that the virus can replicate aggressively. Finally, the "assembly department" puts the copies of the viral genome together with the viral structural proteins, and progeny (many of them—hundreds of thousands, or even millions) are formed, ready to be "shipped" to destinations near and far.

The perfect situation for a virus is to be adapted to an abundant host that is capable of effecting the replication of the virus without becoming compromised or endangered. This would ensure that there is never a lack of a host, and the virus can then continue to do what it does best: replicate.

However, things are not always so perfect. Some viruses actually injure, or even destroy the host they invade. In this instance, the virus is considered a germ. In the history of the world, there have probably been millions of viral germs that have been so destructive to their hosts, that they have caused their own extinction, an evolutionary dead end. In the process, of course, they've killed off their hosts (plants, animals, and people).

How do viruses persist in nature?

Viruses need to be adapted to higher life forms that can function as their hosts, and ensure a stable reservoir of infection in the world; otherwise they would cease to exist. The need for an omnipresent host reservoir is the driving force behind the capacity of viruses to evolve rapidly.

Viral evolution occurs by a number of mechanisms. One is *mutation*.

(I'll discuss this further in the next section.) When a virus mutates, errors occur in the copying of the "wild-type" viral genome. The subsequent gene product proteins are not exact replicas of the genes that spawned them. Instead, they'll have structural changes that confer a selective advantage over those of the "wild-type" virus.

An example, in theory, might be a modification of a viral surface protein that allows a reptile virus (let's imagine a snake flu) to be able to infect a mammal (let's use a skunk). The selective advantage would be a larger reservoir of hosts (snakes and skunks), and a greater likelihood of persistence in nature.

Another method in which a virus may change in the process of selective evolution is through *recombination*. A recombinant virus is one that has adopted genetic material from another virus that has infected the same host. An example would be two different influenza viruses, or perhaps a swine flu virus that is recombinant with a human flu virus. By creating a tapestry of gene products from more than a single virus, the new recombinant virus could acquire qualities that make it better suited to infect specific hosts, or resist immune systems of the new hosts it infects.

How, then, do viruses survive?

The survival of viruses depends upon their ability to reproduce in high numbers within their hosts. They must then efficiently spread to new hosts. Of these, the most successful are those that can infect their hosts without killing them.

For example, the human herpes simplex virus type I (the virus that causes fever blisters) enjoys a prevalence of up to 90 percent in the general population. It persists for the life of its human host, causing unwanted and often embarrassing skin outbreaks, but it doesn't affect the viability of its host. A herpes simplex outbreak will not kill you.

As I said, viruses have proven themselves to be extremely adaptable to a wide array of higher life forms, including plants, bacteria, protozoa, fungi, as well as arthropods, reptiles, and mammals. But how has this astonishing array of viruses survived billions of years of evolutionary change—from the sea, to land, and from overheated volcanic climates to frigid ice ages? How can such simple packets of protein and nucleic acid keep up with the impressive degree of evolutionary change that their more complex hosts have experienced?

The simple answer is that viruses survive by way of their imperfections.

Every time it replicates, various enzymes in the virus cause the host's cells to make copies of the virus. These enzymes are essentially proofreaders of the viral genetic code. However, the proofreading itself is imperfect. In other words, mistakes can happen accidentally. These are the mutations I described in the previous section. The new, mutated virus is subtly different from the virus that spawned it.

As these mutations occur, the copies of the original virus will become different, and more diverse. The more different they are, the more or less infectious they will become for the host's other cells.

In essence, this viral diversification is a highly compressed form of evolution. Instead of evolving over millennia, as humans, animals, and plants do, a virus can evolve over a matter of years, months, days—even hours.

The good news is that spontaneous mutations often cause a higher percentage of biologically ineffective viruses. They'll no longer be able to cause infection, and cease to function.

The bad news is that some other viruses may mutate and escape this biologic dead end, and may have a selective growth advantage due to their unique mutations. In this way, viruses can rapidly adapt to the slower evolutionary changes of their more complex hosts.

For example, the HIV (Human Immunodeficiency Virus) that causes AIDS is a perfect example of how mutations can improve the survival of viral pathogens. This rather simple virus has a short genome, with only 9,718 base pairs. The proofreading enzyme responsible for the HIV virus's replicating, reverse transcriptase, is prone to frequent mistakes. This is an extremely high mutation rate, with about four errors for each copy of virus.

Such errors in duplication can change the virus's ability to destroy immune cells (good news), but it can also make the virus resistant to both the available anti-viral medications and the host's own immune response (bad news).

The HIV virus's high mutation rate is probably the single most important reason why it has reached epidemic proportions around the globe after having jumped from a limited monkey species into people only a few short decades ago. It is also the reason that vaccine development for HIV has been so challenging.

How does a virus replicate?

Once inside your body, the virus has to find a target on whatever kind of host cell it is structurally programmed to invade. This target is the receptor that it can attach or bind to chemically. The virus then breaches the cell membranes and enters the cell proper. The strands of viral genome invade the cell and co-mingle with cell's own genetic material. The virus then co-opts the host cell's enzymatic machinery to transcribe and translate the viral genome into viral-associated proteins. The host cell is now diverted into producing hundreds or thousands of viral copies of the original invader.

When enough viral particles have been produced within the host cell, they are ready to be released. At this stage, the host cell may not survive as its cell membrane is breached and the newly formed virions are released—spewed out by the tens of thousands—to infect other cells in the host.

In other words, host cells are co-opted by the virus's genetic material, reprogrammed to replicate the virus's structural and enzymatic proteins instead of its own, and then they literally cease to exist.

ALL ABOUT THE INFLUENZA VIRUS

As soon as there was recorded history, there were descriptions of influenza.

The word "influenza" was derived from the Italian word for "influence" during the Middle Ages. Back then, disease was more likely to have been thought of as the work of the devil, or carried on the whim of the pre-vailing wind, or "influenced" by astrological configurations.

If only that were true!

Influenza, or the flu, is a respiratory virus. It can't be transmitted through blood (like the Ebola virus) or via an insect bite (like the West Nile virus). The virus binds to the epithelial cells lining the respiratory mucous membranes in your trachea and bronchial tubes.

As the flu virus particles are too small to leave a host on their own, they attach themselves on the host's respiratory secretions—coughs and sneezes and the mucus from runny noses. (These respiratory secretions, or droplets, are usually less than ten micrometers in diameter.) You're likely to be exposed if an infected person sneezes or coughs on you. It's also possible to become infected merely by touching something an in-fected person has just touched, as flu viruses can often survive on sur-faces such as door knobs and elevator buttons for between two and eight hours. They're usually destroyed by sunlight.

As you doubtless know already, the flu is extremely contagious. One of the primary reasons it's so potentially dangerous is that it's usually contagious the day before you're aware that you've got it, and for up to five days after you've gotten sick.

According to the Centers for Disease Control and Prevention (CDC), every year about 5 to 20 percent of Americans get the flu. More than 200,000 people are hospitalized from complications. The annual eco-nomic cost is estimated to be in the range of $10 billion in the United States alone.

Most people do not die from the seasonal flu. The mortality rate is ap-proximately 0.1 percent. About 36,000 people die from the flu each year.

Those killed by the flu are usually the very young, the very old, and the immuno-suppressed from a pre-existing medical condition. They're at the top of each side of a U-shaped curve, with healthy adults at the bottom. (The Spanish Flu did not follow the typical U-shaped curve for fatalities. Most of the deaths occurred in adults in their twenties.) The stress of a systemic viral illness is enough to make them very seriously ill.

Anyone with a pre-existing lung disease will be especially susceptible. If you're already run-down, or extremely exhausted, or malnourished, or a chain smoker, your risk will be higher.

In addition, different viruses may involve cells at different levels, burrowing deeper into tissues. The 1918 Spanish Flu virus was particularly adept at moving extremely quickly into the deepest sections of the lungs, which is one of the reasons it killed so many so quickly. The victims' lungs became so engorged that they were suffocated by their own blood and fluids.

Scarily enough, H5N1 seems to be capable of having a similar effect in its victims.

Of course, being exposed to the flu doesn't automatically mean you'll come down with it. At the beginning of flu season each year (usually in November, as when the weather turns colder, people are more likely to stay indoors, which enhances the possibility of exposure), many people who have no symptoms at all would be surprised to find out they've actually contracted the flu. They're the lucky ones who escaped a few miserable days in bed.

Let's take a look at the influenza virus in more detail.

What is the influenza virus?

The influenza viruses are classified into one of three types (A, B, C), all of which are members of a broader family of viruses called the Orthomyxoviridae.

Influenza B and C viruses generally do not cause pandemics.

Influenza B only infects people. It causes seasonal disease in older adults, very young children, and people with weak immune systems.

Influenza C causes infection in both swine and humans but generally does not cause severe illness.

Influenza A is the major pathogen (disease-causing germ) in humans. It has also used birds, horses, swine, and certain marine life as hosts. The influenza A virus is a diverse group of sub-type viruses that have evolved very efficiently to infect a variety of different hosts. As such, they have been responsible for human pandemics. They are equal opportunity pathogens, as they can infect the very young, the very old, as well as young adults who have healthy immune systems and would normally never succumb to the flu as they did during the 1918 Spanish Flu pandemic.

The genome of the influenza virus is composed of ribonucleic acid (RNA). The RNA provides the code for the structural proteins that form the skeleton of the virus, as well as the proteins that allow the release of the RNA from the viral structure into the host cell.

These viral structural proteins act as antigens, which are substances that the host's immune system sees, and recognizes, as nonhuman or foreign. As a result, antigens trigger the immune response that is designed to prevent, or modify the disease caused by influenza viruses. (For more information, see the next section.)

Influenza viral particles, or virions, are either round or globular in shape. They are incredibly tiny—only about 40 nanometers in diameter. This means that you could fit 250 *million* viral particles positioned side by side on a yardstick. By comparison, a single grain of pollen is one thousand times larger than a single influenza virus.

These influenza particles have knobby-shaped protrusions on their outer surface, composed of two distinct structural proteins, hemagglutinin (the H) and neuraminidase (the N). There are fifteen different H proteins and nine different N proteins, for a possible 135 different subtype combinations.

The H protein is actually a trimer, meaning that it is comprised of three strands of identical proteins. The N protein is a tetramer, with four strands of identical protein. It is the specific structure of the H and the N proteins that are used to classify the subtypes of influenza virus, and which also determine its disease-causing potential. This is of striking importance, as minor changes in the structure of these proteins can account for very different biologic activity, and may mean the difference between a killer virus and a benign virus. I'll discuss this in detail in the next section.

Inside each viral envelope is its genetic material: RNA that codes for eight gene products. The structural H and N proteins dictate the specific appearance of the virus. Structure is also critical to defining which host the virus can infect, and which cells within that host the virus can preferentially invade.

Actually, human viruses are very limited as to which of the hundreds of different cell types they can use to replicate. The hepatitis C virus can only infect liver cells, for example. The herpes simplex virus resides within nerve cells. The AIDS virus preferentially infects a subset of immune lymphocytes, called CD-4, or helper lymphocytes. The influenza group of viruses invades the respiratory tract lining cells, called the epithelial lining cells of the trachea and bronchial tubes. To a large extent, the preferred cell type determines what kind of illness the infected host experiences, and what kind of immune defense it mounts.

What are influenza A viruses?

There are three main types of influenza A causing human disease from year to year: H1N1, H1N2, and H3N2. The Spanish Flu of 1918 was an H1N1 virus.

From one year to the next, these viral subtypes cause seasonal outbreaks and epidemics. If there were no changes in the type of influenza virus affecting the human population, infections with this germ would quickly cease. That is because immunity to the viruses would develop among an increasing percentage of the world population. Once a critical number of immune persons are present within the population, the virus would no longer be able to replicate. It will, to put it simply, run out of hosts. No host means no replication. End of virus.

However, the influenza virus has acquired the ability to overcome this challenge by our immune systems. It does this through what's termed "antigenic variation."

With antigenic variation, the influenza virus is capable of changing its structure. When that happens, it can evade the protection of the host's immune response without compromising its capacity to cause disease. It remains fully able to keep on replicating and keep on causing disease.

With influenza A, antigenic changes involve the structural H (hemagglutinin) and N (neuraminidase) proteins. Antigenic variation may be minor (antigenic *drift*), or major (antigenic *shift*).

With antigenic drift, minor changes in the H protein, for example, will not change its structure enough to warrant a new subtype designation. An

H2 virus will remain an H2. But, the host's antibodies, whose function in the body is to inactivate the virus, *do* perceive the changes. This is a new situation for them. They may not be as effective in suppressing the virus as they might have been had the H protein not undergone a drift.

As discussed earlier, this chameleonlike ability to change itself is the reason that influenza persists in the human population, and why we have been unable to rid ourselves of this germ.

Actually, it is remarkable that the influenza A virus is able to undergo antigenic drift so quickly within the population. From year to year, minor changes in the amino acid structure of the H proteins can be detected—explaining why a new flu shot is needed every year. These remarkably small variations change the virus's pathogenicity, or its ability to cause human disease.

It is also remarkable that despite the myriad of possible mutations, there are rarely more than several variants in the population at any one time. This is why it is possible to protect a large percentage of the population from seasonal influenza using an annual trivalent vaccine. (See chapter 7 for more about vaccines.)

Antigenic shift is another matter altogether.

With an antigenic shift, there are such major changes in the structure of the H and N proteins that they bear no similarity whatsoever to previous viral strains. Our bodies' immune systems see that these new viruses are totally novel germs. We have no immunity to them. We are utterly unable to defend ourselves immunologically against these new, shifted subtypes.

As such, when a new virus subtype caused by an antigenic shift is discovered, it is often the warning sign of impending pandemics.

The 1889 flu pandemic was caused by an H2N2 virus.

The 1918 pandemic was caused by an antigenically shifted virus, H1N1.

That in turn shifted in 1957 back toH2N2.

Which evolved into the H3N2 virus in 1968.

How does influenza A virus cause disease? How does our immune system respond?

The influenza A virus isn't lethal on its own. Generally speaking, viruses can only invade a limited repertoire of cells. During that time, your

HOW DO ANTIBODIES WORK?

Technically speaking, the humoral immune response is orchestrated by B-lymphocytes. They produce antibodies that bind to viral antigens (the viral structural proteins). Antibodies are mounted against the H (hemagglutinin) and the N (neuraminidase) surface proteins of the virus, as well as a number of other viral-associated proteins.

It takes about seven to fourteen days for these lymphocyte antibodies to appear after the primary influenza A infection. They remain measurable in your body for years. If you are re-exposed to the same, or related, strains of virus, there will be a brisk antibody response, with large quantities of the lymphocytes appearing very rapidly. (To get even more technical, antibodies are produced locally in the form of a surface antibody, secretory IgA, which lies in wait and inactivates the virus before it has a chance to invade the respiratory epithelial cells during a subsequent infection. Antibodies of different classes [IgG, IgM, and IgA] are also produced systemically, and travel in the bloodstream to arrive at the site of infection.)

As these antibodies are highly protective against specific subtypes of the influenza A virus, you would *not* become reinfected with a strain for which you already have antibodies present. Most important, antibodies to one strain of influenza A may be highly, or partially protective against related strains that have undergone antigenic drift. (Yet another reason to get a flu shot—the more antibodies you have to different strains of the flu, the more likely you will have some immune response to subsequent related strains.)

body's functions remain relatively normal—until your body recognizes it has been invaded.

That's when an immune system response kicks into action. As with other viral infections, the body's immune response to influenza A infection involves all components of the immune system.

Another arm of the immune response is the cellular immune response. This arm of the immune system invokes lymphocytes that produce chemicals with a generalized anti-viral activity (such as interferon), and as cytokines, that are designed to modulate and regulate the body's immune response. In addition, cytotoxic lymphocytes are killer cells that can seek out infected host cells and destroy them, which limits the ability of the

DOES HAVING THE FLU GIVE YOU
ANY IMMUNITY TO NEW STRAINS?

Remember, the flu virus is a perfect parasite. It has to find a host, spreading from person to person—or else it would be permanently eradicated. In order to keep that from happening, a small degree of influenza will always exist throughout the year, in every corner of the globe.

The World Health Organization (WHO) is responsible for trying to predict the annual, seasonal strains of influenza. It has its own global surveillance system in place, tracking the predominate strains. They do this by examining the virus's genetic material, and by doing so are able to recognize the antigenic drift from year to year. They make an educated guess about what strains are likely to hit, then relay this information to vaccine manufacturers, who need months to develop the coming year's supply.

Even if you get a flu shot, there's no guarantee that you're still not going to get some kind of flu virus. Influenza viruses mutate so quickly that no one is ever going to be totally immune to them. In addition, older strains of flu viruses that have disappeared for years can return with a vengeance once the immunity to them has died out.

Once you've had a particular strain of flu, your immune response remains protective against that specific strain for some time. We're not able to pinpoint this time frame with precision, but it is probably several years or more. We're also not able to *prove* that immunity to a specific strain gives any immunity to other strains, but we think it does.

Some researchers believe that a variant of the lethal H1N1 virus that caused the Spanish Flu pandemic had been circulating decades before, explaining why relatively few older people (usually the first victims of flu) died from the 1918 version. If this is true, their immunity would have persisted for many years. A pandemic or epidemic requires a large number of susceptible (non-immune) people, and epidemics and pandemics end once there are fewer non-immune people in the population. No hosts, no virus.

virus to replicate effectively. The cytotoxic lymphocyte response peaks after fourteen days. Of course, if you've gotten a flu shot to the strain in question, you'll already have antibodies to it, and your body will mount an effective assault on the virus particles and be able to destroy them before they have a chance to invade your host cells and replicate. If you take an established anti-viral treatment such as Tamiflu as soon as there are any symptoms, it can also interfere with the virus to keep it from replicating.

Bottom line: It takes time for any human body that has not already been vaccinated for the specific strain of influenza A to mount a major, maximum offensive against a flu virus attack—anywhere from one to two weeks. This inescapable biological fact means that you will have little immune system protection from a highly aggressive strain of the flu, such as H5N1.

So that explains why I feel so crummy when I have the flu?

Exactly. With influenza A, the virus enters through the mucous membranes of the nose, eyes, and oral cavity and invades the upper respiratory tract lining cells (the respiratory epithelial cells). Once the virus has "docked" with the cell surface, the process of viral entry and viral replication begin. If unchecked (by an anti-viral medication), the process cannot be undone once it has started. A viral invasion into the host cell means the end of life for the cell.

So, when you have the flu, the respiratory epithelial cells invaded and co-opted by the flu virus will die—but only after hundreds or thousands of influenza A progeny have been released to invade surrounding cells. This is the trigger for an immune system attack on the invader, setting in motion a cascade of inflammatory responses by your own immune cells and disease-fighting antibodies.

An easy way to picture this is if you trip on the sidewalk and sprain your ankle. It swells up and is incredibly painful. The inflammation is your body's natural response to this injury, and its function is to repair something that's been ripped, torn, or bruised in some way. You need this inflammation to help you heal, but in the meantime, you can't walk on your ankle without screaming in agony.

With a virus, the inflammatory response happens *throughout* your body. Having a fever, chills, aches, and the blahs are the internal equivalent of that swollen ankle. These symptoms are caused by the cytokines and cytotoxic lymphocytes—not by the virus.

If your inflammatory response to a virus becomes too severe, however, you could be in serious trouble. Blood vessels dilate, to help increase the cellular traffic to the site of infection, and the result is a fever. Lymphocytes and other mononuclear cells also respond to the area, causing further congestion and tissue disruption. The increased traffic causes body fluids to leave the blood vessels and accumulate within the tissues themselves. This fluid is otherwise known as mucus. It leaves your body after it has clogged your nasal cavity and/or upper airway, resulting in the well-known sinus misery (or catarrh).

If the influenza virus invades the lower respiratory tract, however, fluids accumulate in the lungs, interfering with the exchange of oxygen. This causes pneumonia, and is frequently lethal. A person can die from the flu when enough of the respiratory epithelial cells are killed by the invading virus, and when the body's immune response is overall too intense. If that happens, the lungs are flooded with blood and fluids and suffocation results.

In addition, some flu sufferers who survive the initial viral infection and subsequent immune response become ill from secondary bacterial infections that prey upon the body's weakened state. (For more, see the section on bacteria on page 51.)

As I mentioned in chapter 1, the virus that caused the Spanish Flu pandemic of 1918 was more virulent than the seasonal flu in a number of important ways. As it was a new strain in the affected population, there were no preexisting (secretory IgA) antibodies to it, and so the H1N1 virus was able to invade respiratory epithelial cells unimpeded by an immune response. Furthermore, this specific virus was somehow able to reach down to the deeper portions of the lung quite quickly after the initial infection, thereby causing life-threatening pneumonia in a majority of those who became ill. Also unusual was the fact that the H1N1 strain of influenza appeared able to invade cells in organ systems other than the respiratory tract. The cellular devastation stretched beyond the lungs to involve the heart, gastrointestinal tract, and the nervous system.

In addition, this virus was able to speed up the normal dying process in cells. Every cell in the body is pre-programmed to die after a certain time. That's totally normal, as it's needed to make way for new cells. During the 1918 pandemic, the virus replicated so quickly, and provoked such an intense immune system response, that it killed with incredible speed.

Not only that, but the 1918 strain also became superefficient at infecting one host after another—people spreading the virus to other people. Remember that a perfect parasite has to adapt itself to a specific host so it can replicate. If a virus is too efficient, it will kill too many or all of its hosts.

Within about thirteen months, the H1N1 strain disappeared. It had no human hosts left to infect. Had it been less lethal, it could have mutated into a longer lasting, more benign state in order to survive.

Can the H5N1 avian virus become a human virus?

The answer is yes, but not without some changes.

The H5N1 avian influenza A virus has infected poultry, ducks, and other migratory birds, and has also been transmitted to tigers, cats, and pigs. To date, the virus has not demonstrated any of the 1918 Spanish Flu's agility in infecting (and killing) people. We know this, because the only people who've been infected since 1997, when the first H5N1 cases were detected in Asia, were bird handlers who most likely had extensive exposure to the virus. There may have been one or two cases of secondary human-to-human transmission, but that is not yet certain. The good news is that after seven years, the H5N1 virus that has been wreaking havoc in the poultry population has, as yet, not been able to do the same in humans.

So, what would it take for H5N1 to become a virus with higher proclivity for human hosts, like the H1N1 virus of 1918? It would probably have to evolve into a different virus.

But don't take too much comfort in that statement. There are many different influenza A virus subtypes and strains co-existing in the world, in a wide array of animal hosts. Viral evolution, as I've already mentioned, can occur over very short periods of time, in three different ways.

1. The H5N1 currently residing in birds—they represent the major reservoir right now—could mutate on its own, and jump into humans as a more virulent strain. Just like that.
2. An intermediary host, such as swine, could serve as the melting pot in which the viral genes that encode for virulence in people are recombined. The result would be a much more dangerous human virus.

   Pigs have served as intermediary hosts before. If a pig became infected with both a bird virus and a human virus at the same time, the new viral strain could be unique in its propensity to infect and kill human hosts. A recent study sponsored by the National Institute of Allergy and Infectious Diseases (NIAID), a division of the National Institutes of Health (NIH), conducted at the University of Iowa Center for Emerging Infectious Diseases, found that pig farmers, veterinarians, and meat processors who routinely come into contact with pigs in their jobs have a markedly increased risk of infection with the flu viruses that infect pigs.

   "Pigs play a role in transmitting influenza virus to humans," says NIAID director Anthony S. Fauci, M.D. "The worry is that if a pig were to become simultaneously infected with both a human and an avian influenza virus, genes from these viruses could reassemble into a new virus that could be transmitted to and cause disease in people."

   The study's co-director, Dr. Gregory Gray, added, "If migratory birds introduce the H5N1 bird flu virus into swine or poultry populations in this country, agricultural workers may be at a much greater risk of developing a variant H5N1 and passing it along to nonagricultural workers."
3. The H5N1 virus could acquire these virulence factors directly from human hosts that become co-infected with both bird and human strains of influenza A. The new influenza virus could, for example, have recombined bird-type H with a human-type N.

These are extremely sobering scenarios to ponder. They aren't futuristic science fiction scenarios. They're *distinct* possibilities.

While the creation of a pandemic strain of the flu depends upon a large number of chance events coming together in a very precise order, remember the billions of birds and pigs and people on this planet, and the trillions upon trillions of viral particles that are all interacting at this very moment.

It is not so much a question of *will* another pandemic occur, but *when.*

Will viruses ever be totally eradicated?

The answer is no, and that is probably a good thing. Of course, we wish that some viruses, like the bird flu—which, so far at least, are poorly adapted and lethal to their incidental human hosts—could be eradicated.

Viruses should not be thought of as uniformly destructive, however. Given the fact that they have successfully cohabited the planet with all other forms of life for billions of years, we must assume that they serve important roles in the overall bio-ecology of our world.

In the modern medical world, we use viruses in various laboratory diagnostic and research endeavors. Many of our most successful vaccines have been derived from viruses (see chapter 7 for more information). And viruses will play a part in the future of medical miracles that may to a large extent rely on gene therapy. Diseases such as hemophilia and rare metabolic disorders are caused by human gene mutations that deprive those that are afflicted with them of critical gene products. Viruses that are benign to human hosts may someday soon become the delivery vehicles of these missing genes. Instead of aggressively assaulting, invading, and killing the host cells, they will be able to gently invade healthy cells and deliver the missing genetic material into the human genome. A similar approach is being explored for potential AIDS vaccines, which may eventually save millions of lives.

Viruses in nature probably also control other potential germs. For example, bacteriophages, which are viruses that infect bacteria, may control the growth of potentially deadly bacteria.

And let's put viruses into evolutionary perspective. Human beings have evolved over hundreds of thousands to millions of years. Viruses have certainly preceded us. Over *billions* of years, those infinitesimal virus particles have acquired the ability to adapt to ever-changing environments.

Viruses are such remarkable entities that they can evolve over months . . . or weeks . . . even *hours*. Who do you think has the advantage?

As medical science currently stands, it can respond to viral threats only *after* they are recognized. Hopefully, we will have gained experience and expertise that will allow us to anticipate and intervene effectively, and limit human suffering.

WHAT IS THE DIFFERENCE BETWEEN VIRUSES AND BACTERIA?

During the lethal Spanish Flu pandemic of 1918, many millions who survived the initial stages of the H1N1 viral infection died from the secondary bacterial infections that preyed upon their weakened state. So, bacteria are a crucial link in our understanding and treatment of influenza.

What is a bacteria?

A bacteria is a single-celled living germ.

Comparing a virus to a bacteria is tantamount to comparing a boomerang to a snake. One is inanimate. The other is alive. Both, of course, can kill you if you happen to get in their way.

Basically, bacteria have a number of components that viruses don't have. They have cell walls and cell membranes, and a nucleus inside, as well as mitochondria, which are little organelles that have metabolic activity and produce the energy needed for all the cell's functions. They respire, and they also replicate in a process called binary fission, in which they split into two identical copies. They can do this within an extremely short time span, usually within a few hours (and sometimes less). They also have their own genetic material, which is the substrate upon which it replicates itself.

A virus, being inanimate, can't produce energy. It can only replicate.

Not all bacteria cause disease. Our bodies have developed what are called commensal relationships with certain beneficial bacteria. They help our bodies break down products, digest food in our intestines, and make vitamins, such as Vitamin K. Some of these beneficial bacteria occupy certain niches within our bodies or on our skin that actually keep more virulent bacteria out of the picture. That's called bacterial interference.

Our bodies are walking petri dishes full of bacteria. Our mouths, for example, are full of germs that don't normally cause disease—unless there's some sort of extenuating circumstance. If the dentist has to pull a tooth, leaving you with a gaping hole in your gums, a localized (and easily treated) socket infection might ensue. If your daughter skins her knee on the playground, it can get infected. Or if your immune system is weak in some way that alters the balance between the commensal organisms and the host, you can get a severe bacterial infection as well.

What are the treatments for bacterial infections?

Since bacteria are alive, the way to treat them is to kill them.

Antibiotics are medications that function by interfering with the bacteria's metabolic functions. Different antibiotics run different kinds of interference. Penicillin will inhibit the growth of or cause a disruption in the bacteria's cell wall as it's replicating, so it can't keep on doing what it wants to do and it dies off. Other antibiotics actually get into the bacterial cells and kill the bacteria by interfering with the process of protein synthesis.

As a virus is not alive, antibiotics will have no effect on it. Most people are unaware of this fact—we live in a pill-popping culture where people expect (if not demand) a quick fix to every disease. Manufacturers of disinfectant products that claim to "kill viruses" would be more precise if they stated that their products "inactivated viruses." In addition, many of my patients theoretically understand that antibiotics are not prescribed for viruses, but that doesn't stop them from asking for them.

This is a tremendous problem for physicians, and for the public's health in general. Certain strains of bacteria that had been instantly obliterated by antibiotics years ago have since become drug-resistant. Bacteria evolve just as viruses do. That means a germ that had been easily treatable might now be lethal. Should there be a flu pandemic, thousands if not millions of people may become susceptible to secondary bacterial infections after surviving the initial viral assault. If they can't be treated successfully with antibiotics, they will die from diseases that should not have killed them.

There's never any reason to take an antibiotic unless your physician directly indicates it for a specific condition. Always finish the prescription even if you feel better, because if you don't, the weaker bacteria will be killed but the more potent bacteria will be able to survive, and possibly evolve into something more ferocious.

Don't forget that antibiotics often have unpleasant side effects. One of the most common is the destruction of much of the beneficial bacteria that live inside our intestines. Every time you pop an antibiotic, you're exposing the entire microbiota that live inside of you to unnecessary termination. Be sure to take a pro-biotic supplement of acidophilus and bifidus (two of the beneficial intestinal bacteria) whenever you take any antibiotics for more than a few days.

Chapter 3.

A BIRD FLU PRIMER

Now that you know about human viruses and bacteria, let's take a look at the bird flu virus.

ALL ABOUT BIRD FLU

What is bird flu?

Bird flu, or avian influenza, is a highly contagious virus. It can affect domesticated chickens, turkeys, pheasants, quail, ducks, geese, guinea fowl, as well as other varieties of birds, including migratory waterfowl. Pigs and horses can be infected, too.

Domesticated flocks of chickens and turkeys seem to be the most susceptible to bird flu. Wild migratory birds, such as ducks, can be carriers without seeming to develop any symptoms. They don't get sick at all despite high-grade infection. Avian influenza is extremely well adapted to its avian hosts.

All animals can suffer from viruses causing the flu. In 1988, there was a harbor seal epidemic in Denmark's Wadden Sea, where an H7N7 virus wiped out about 20 percent of the harbor seal population and rendered them near to extinction. (Luckily, that strain was not transmissible to humans. Its structure made it poorly adapted to human host cells.)

Are there different strains of bird flu?

There are many, many kinds of bird flu, and two strains of them: low pathogenic (LPAI—Low Pathogenic Avian Influenza), which usually is mild or asymptomatic; and high pathogenic (HPAI—High Pathogenic Avian Influenza), which is almost always fatal to birds.

As with human flu, some of the birds infected with LPAI can get very sick and die—but they don't spread disease to people. According to Dr. Ron DeHaven, an administrator with the Animal and Plant Health Inspection Service (APHIS) of the U.S. Department of Agriculture, "LPAI has been identified in the United States and indeed around the world since the early 1900s, and is a relatively common finding—just as human flu viruses are a common finding in people."

Dr. Jim Clark of the Canadian Food Inspection Agency said that a variant of the H5 virus is likely to be found in at least 7 percent of all wild birds in North America at any given time. Not the killer H5N1, but in a less virulent form that is not transmissible to people.

But, on the other hand, H5N1, the current cause for concern, is a highly pathogenic subtype, an HPAI. That's where the problem lies. Only the H5 and H7 subtypes have ever been shown to be highly pathogenic to *both* birds and people.

As you learned in the previous chapter, viruses have H (hemagglutinin) and N (neuraminidase) proteins on their surface. There are fifteen different H proteins and nine different N proteins, for a possible 135 different subtype combinations. Each combination is a different subtype.

Human flu is divided into A, B, and C types; only A and B can kill people, as I also discussed in the previous chapter. All known subtypes of flu A viruses can be found in birds, so it's a fair assumption that some of the genetic material in the human influenza A virus originated in birds.

In other words, bird flu and human flu come from the same family of viruses, and bird flu is the original cause of all human influenza "Type

A" viruses. Most strains of bird flu have been around for as long as there've been birds—hundreds of millions of years. This particular type of bird-related illness was first recognized as a specific disease in Italy in 1878, although scientists at the time did not yet know what a virus was.

Of all these different strains, which ones can infect people?

Only four of the avian subtypes can infect and sicken people: H5N1, H7N7, H7N3, and H9N2. Most of the other strains usually do not pose any significant health risk to people.

How does bird flu spread in the avian population?

The bird flu is shed in animal saliva, nasal secretions, and, unlike human influenza, feces. It spreads when wild, migratory birds, attracted by food, fly down and land in the barnyard to scavenge through the flock's feed. Or when wild birds and domesticated birds share a water source.

According to the U.S. Department of Agriculture, "In an agricultural setting, animal manure containing influenza virus can contaminate dust and soil, causing infection when the contaminated dust is inhaled. Contaminated farm equipment, feed, cages, or shoes can carry the virus from farm to farm. The virus can also be carried on the bodies and feet of animals, such as rodents. The virus can remain infectious at cool temperatures, in contaminated manure, for at least three months. In water, the virus can survive for up to four days at 72°F and more than 30 days at 32°F."

Bird flu can also spread when infected birds are transported—to the slaughterhouse or to markets.

How quickly does the H5N1 virus spread from infected poultry to other poultry?

It can spread like wildfire. Most commercially farmed chickens live in enormous buildings, sometimes the size of football fields, in extremely close proximity to tens of thousands of other chickens. It's an ideal environment in which a virus can begin to mutate and spread.

H5N1 is so virulent that chickens which have gotten sick in the morning can be dead by the evening. And this strain has an almost 100 percent mortality rate in commercially reared poultry.

During a HPAI outbreak in the Netherlands in February 2003, the weather was unusually dry and the winds unusually strong. Infected dirt and dust quickly swirled from one farm to another. In addition, after the infected, dying, and dead chickens were being destroyed, their carcasses were swiftly removed and properly disposed of, but their litter, manure, and feed were not. Until all the contaminated surfaces and feed were cleaned up, they could remain contagious.

In October 2005, *Nature* magazine sent a reporter to a street market in Shanghai, China, where plucked chickens were on sale right next to other vendors hawking fruit and vegetables. Most worrisome, chicken vendors applied the age-old technique of proving a bird's health by holding it upside down to inspect its rear end for "pinkness." There's only one way to move aside the feathers and other debris to do so—by blowing on them. And as chickens aren't exactly in the habit of practicing bathroom etiquette after they do their business, there will always be some amount of fecal matter in the area.

Since bird flu viruses are spread via feces, this is an ideal method of spewing virus over a large area.

Doubtless these vendors might stop their blow-and-show routine if they knew that H5N1 is so lethal to birds that a single gram of contaminated manure can contain enough virus to infect one million birds.

That's a very little bit of virus, and a very lot of dead chickens.

How is bird flu treated in birds?

Bird flu is so lethal that there is no treatment for it once birds in a flock are infected and becoming ill. The only way to manage an outbreak is to destroy the entire flock. Often, neighboring flocks are destroyed as well, in an effort to contain the spread of the virus.

Thankfully, there is a bird flu vaccine—but only for birds. It is very effective protection against the H5N1 strain in Asia. (For more information about vaccines, see chapter 7.)

In a national bird flu vaccine bank run by the APHIS, two types of vaccines are stored: 20 million doses of H5 and 20 million doses of H7.

H7 is not a threat to people; it's the Low Pathogen Avian Influenza (LPAI) strain. However, it's prudent to keep a vaccine for it on hand, as H7 may some day mutate into a High Pathogen Avian Influenza (HPAI) like H5N1.

Have other animal viruses infected people before?

Yes. West Nile virus is a perfect example. We were able to track the first entry from a person who got on a plane in 1999 in Israel and landed in New York. From there, we could see the disease spread westward with incredible speed.

People can also be infected by swine flu, from pigs. Although it rarely causes symptoms in pigs or people, in 1976, one soldier training at Fort Dix in New Jersey contracted swine flu and died, and a nationwide panic ensued. (See chapter 5 for more about swine flu.)

How does bird flu spread to people?

With only a few possible exceptions, the H5N1 bird flu virus has so far infected only those who've had some kind of close contact with poultry—either through their work on farms, or in markets, or by killing, plucking the feathers, and handling a chicken or duck, which brings hands and feet into close contact with feces, mucus, and infected tissues. This close handling of recently infected and killed poultry prior to cooking spreads the virus—not the consuming of the cooked animal itself.

One of the primary reasons the H5N1 virus originated in Asia is that millions of families there live in close proximity to their farm animals. These animals usually don't live in barns, but in penned yards right next to homes. They often wander into these homes and play areas where children are likely to handle either infected birds or contaminated soil that is teeming with virus-laden chicken excrement.

And because subsistence farmers in Asia need their poultry flocks as food for their families, they are not likely to cull their flocks if a chicken gets sick—not unless they're instructed and then forced to do so by local officials (and sometimes not even then, especially if it's a question of feeding their families or starving). They're likely to sell the sick birds, or to eat them. Many millions of people living in isolated communities, with no electricity and certainly no Internet, have no idea that the H5N1 bird flu even exists, or that it may become transmissible on a larger scale to people. This is a huge public health issue.

Apart from H5N1, have other bird flu viruses ever infected people?

Yes. I'll discuss this in the next chapter.

What is the biggest difference between human flu and the H5N1 bird flu?

What's scary about the H5N1 strain is that it seems to be more virulent than most other strains. The H5N1 strain causes pneumonia to develop, by affecting the lower reaches of the respiratory tract much earlier than normal. It also possesses the ability to invade human cells in organs *other* than those that seasonal influenza can invade—namely, the heart, liver, and the central nervous system. (This factor is similar to one in the 1918 pandemic's H1N1 virus, which likely explains why so many victims later developed encephalitis and Parkinson's disease.)

For these reasons, H5N1 is quite difficult to cure. Those unlucky enough to have been infected by the bird flu have had typical symptoms—fever, cough, sore throat, shortness of breath, muscle aches, and lethargy. Some develop conjunctivitis (irritation of the lining of the eye). Others have progressed to pneumonia and acute respiratory distress syndrome (ARDS).

SURVIVING BIRD FLU

As reported by the BBC (British Broadcasting Corporation) in February 2005, a forty-two-year-old Vietnamese salesman named Nguyen Thanh Hung was infected by the bird flu—and lived to talk about it. His brother Nguyen Hung Viet was not so fortunate.

The brothers had both eaten their favorite dish, "tiet canh," made with congealed raw duck blood and herbs at a family dinner. The duck in question had appeared perfectly healthy.

A day later, Viet ran a fever, and rapidly worsened. He was tested for bird flu, initially with negative results. Hung nursed him until he died a week later. The next day, Hung developed a fever, and found it hard to breathe. He went to a clinic, where he was put in quarantine. "My concern grew each day, as my temperature was staying extremely high," he said. "At the worst moment, two-thirds of one lung was severely affected. Still, when the doctors told me I had bird flu I was totally shocked. I knew nothing about it and it scared me. The test on the specimen taken from my brother also came back that day, as positive. I got into such a panic, even though my fever was beginning to subside. For two nights, I didn't sleep. I told myself I should not doze off at any point—something may happen inside me, inside my brain, and I may never wake up."

Luckily, Hung pulled through. Even though he may have handled and had eaten the same raw duck blood dish as his brother, which presumably provided the same exposure to the H5N1 pathogen, local officials still worried that his was the second suspected case of human-to-human bird flu transmission in Vietnam. Hung had not sickened at the same time as his brother, and had spent countless hours nursing him and being further exposed to the virus.

When he was investigating the current outbreak, Secretary of Health and Human Services Michael Leavitt met with another Vietnamese family, the Sons, who also survived bird flu. Leavitt relayed this story to the National Press Club in a talk on pandemic preparedness in October 2005.

At the Sons' home, the chickens were stacked seven deep in cages behind their home. When five of their three hundred chickens got sick, they decided to eat some of the others, so the loss of their flock wouldn't be a total disaster. A week later, Mr. Son got sick.

"First, it was nausea, then fever and a cough. 'It seemed routine,' he said. 'I have experienced it all before.' Two hours passed; suddenly, everything worsened. Excruciating pain coursed along his rib cage.

" 'Every cough,' he said, 'was like coughing up my lungs.'

"He described his condition as 'completely losing control.' He was losing the capacity to breathe. Two hours after that, their four-year-old girl became ill with the same symptoms."

As with Nguyen Thanh Hung, the Sons were lucky to have survived.

What saved them was treatment with anti-viral medication (see chapter 8).

Not only is the H5N1 virus devastatingly lethal to chickens, but it has a staggeringly high mortality rate in the people it has made ill—nearly 50 percent. No other epidemic or pandemic of human flu has ever killed such a high percentage of its victims.

How are people infected with H5N1 treated?

The H5N1 virus in Asia is treated with anti-viral medications: oseltamavir (Tamiflu) and zanamavir (Relenza). The bad news is that in June 2005, the WHO reported that the bird flu was resistant to older, low-cost anti-viral drugs commonly used to treat the flu, amantadine (Symmatrel) and rimantadine (Flumadine). This may be due to overuse by Chinese farmers who added the older class of anti-virals to chicken feed.

If H5N1 manages to develop resistance to Tamiflu and Relenza, we're in big trouble, as there are currently no other anti-viral medications available to combat it. For more information about anti-viral medications, see chapter 8.

There is as yet no vaccine that can be given to people as a preventative measure for the H5N1 virus. The National Institutes of Health (NIH) is currently is overseeing clinical trials of an experimental vaccine. These trials began in April 2005. For more information about the flu vaccine, see chapter 7.

Can you get bird flu from raw chicken or duck?

Yes. The World Health Organization reported a study in which H5N1 was discovered in imported frozen duck meat. Poultry bought from live markets, which may appear healthy when purchased but are in fact incubating the virus, can spread it when killed, plucked, and handled. Any kind of food prepared with raw poultry blood can be contaminated. Eggs from infected poultry might be as well.

For now, you should stay away from any live poultry markets in Asia or any other countries where H5N1 has appeared, and you should take extra precautions when handling any raw poultry in affected areas. (See chapter 9 for more information.)

Also, for now, if you do not work in the poultry industry, you can be exposed to the H5N1 virus *only* when handling infected raw poultry. You cannot catch bird flu from cooked chicken or duck, or from cooked eggs. To be on the safe side, be certain to cook all poultry and eggs thoroughly. Do not taste batter or any other food if made with raw eggs. (These are normal precautions for the avoidance of salmonella contamination from raw eggs.)

Is there any evidence at this time that the H5N1 virus currently circulating in Asia is in our country, either in birds or in people?

No, although it may very well be here, and we just haven't found it—yet.

But even if it's here, I still can't get bird flu from birds—right?

Unless you're a poultry worker or live in close proximity to and handle raw poultry in the Asian countries where there've been cases of bird-to-person transmission. So far that appears to be correct.

Let's say you're visiting New York, and you stop to eat a hot dog on a bench in Central Park, admiring the passersby and the natural beauty of the greenery around you. This being New York, it also means annoyingly aggressive New York pigeons, known for their uncanny ability to spot a hot-dog-bun crumb the second it hits the sidewalk. These pigeons might be annoying, especially when they leave their poop near your shoes. But although the bird flu can be transmitted via bird feces, pigeons in New York are not hosts for H5N1 virus. They will not give you avian flu.

If the bird flu virus mutates into a virus that is transmissible from person to person, you still won't have to worry about the pigeons in Central Park. They won't make you sick. Other *people* will.

Part III

THE CURRENT SITUATION

Chapter 4.

H5N1 IS *on* *the* MOVE

H5N1 IS ON THE MOVE

"Fish gotta swim and birds gotta fly" go the lyrics of that wonderful Gershwin song, "Can't Help Lovin' That Man of Mine."

Too bad that birds gotta fly right now, because they're flying all over the world, carrying H5N1 with them.

Let's take a look at when and where the problem with H5N1 began.

When did the infectious disease community begin to get alarmed about H5N1?

Ground Zero for H5N1 was in Hong Kong, in 1997.

For the first time ever, this specific virus was transmitted directly from birds to people. This transmission was not expected, and it was certainly not welcome news for public health officials.

Nor was it welcome news for several hundred people. Of these, eighteen people were hospitalized. Six of them died.

Even scarier, one of the cases may have been a person-to-person transmission between family members. The other seventeen had been transmitted from chickens to people. As a result, over 1.5 million chickens were killed to try and contain the virus.

At the time, the culling of so many chickens seemed to have worked. No new cases appeared.

Until six years later.

In 2003, again in Hong Kong, H5N1 appeared in two members of a family who had recently traveled to China. One survived, the other died. How and where precisely they'd been infected was never determined.

And then the real problems started. WHO has since classified this as the first wave of this outbreak.

- At the end of 2003, WHO reported that two tigers and two leopards in a Thai zoo died from H5N1 after eating infected chicken carcasses—the first time it had ever appeared in big cats.
- By mid-December, 2003 through early February, 2004, outbreaks of H5N1 began to be reported in Vietnam and Thailand, as well as in Korea, Japan, Cambodia, Laos, Indonesia, and China. The number of chickens involved was staggering. More than *100 million* chickens either died from the virus or were killed in an attempt to prevent its spread.
- At the same time, several human deaths from H5N1 were reported in Vietnam and Thailand.

By March 2004, local officials gave a huge sigh of relief. They thought they'd eradicated H5N1 from the poultry population. Twenty-three people in Vietnam had become infected; sixteen of them died. In Thailand, eight of the twelve people infected died. No more human cases appeared.

They were wrong. By the end of June 2005, H5N1 was back with a vengeance—in Vietnam, Thailand, Cambodia, Laos, China, and Indonesia. (Korea, Japan, and Malaysia appeared to have contained this outbreak, so far.)

This was the beginning of the second phase. Worse, H5N1 was more lethal than ever.

- An outbreak at a nature preserve at Qinghai Lake in northwest China in April 2005, eventually killed 6,345 wild fowl, which had previously thought to have been immune to H5N1. Researchers theorized that migratory wild fowl could continue to spread the virus around the world on their upcoming winter flight paths. This was extremely worrisome. (In the last century, there have only been two previous "die-offs" caused by High Pathogenic Avian Influenza [HPAI] in migratory birds—H5N3 in South Africa in 1961, and H5N1 in Hong Kong in 2002–2003.)

• In May, H5N1 was found in pigs in Indonesia, and has since been found in pigs in China. Remember that in 1918, the bird flu was thought to have traveled from birds to pigs to people. While infecting mammals such as pigs, the virus can swap genes with preexisting human flu strains already present in the pigs. Not a good eventuality.

• By August, three more people in Vietnam were infected. All three died. Then, H5N1 was detected in birds in Siberia, Tibet, and Kazakhstan.

• In September, there were fatal human cases in Indonesia. Four people in Cambodia had already died, too.

• In October, there were confirmed cases in birds and poultry in Mongolia, Romania, Turkey, Croatia, and on the Greek island of Chios. Smuggled Chinese birds infected with H5N1 were confiscated in Taiwan and quarantined. A sole infected parrot imported into the United Kingdom had the virus, too. A total of six provinces in China have reported nine different outbreaks in poultry and birds.

The fact that bird flu has appeared in Europe makes it likely to spread on the wings of migratory birds into the Middle East and Africa.

• In the middle of November, three cases had been identified in China, with two fatalities.

• By December 2005, bird flu appeared in the Ukraine. A five-year-old boy died in Thailand, and two more cases were reported in China.

Since H5N1 first went on the warpath in 2003, over 150 million birds have died—either from the virus itself or from having to have been destroyed.

As this book went to press in January 2006, there were 74 deaths and 142 infected people in Cambodia, China, Indonesia, Thailand, and Vietnam.

Is H5N1 likely to come to America?

Those birds that gotta fly, well, they gotta fly over North America, too.

For most of us tracking the progress of H5N1, the answer to this question isn't *if* but *when*.

There are several ways the bird flu virus might come to America.

Migrating Wildfowl

H5N1 probably won't enter our borders in a shipment of frozen chicken from China. It will enter on the wings of migrating birds.

OUTBREAKS OF OTHER BIRD FLU VIRUSES IN PEOPLE OUTSIDE OF THE UNITED STATES

As you know by now, bird flu viruses are extremely common—in birds. In the last few years, there have been several outbreaks of *other* bird flu viruses that have indeed infected people. Luckily, there have only been a handful of cases, and a lone fatality. Here's a brief list:

- H9N2 (Low Pathogenic Avian Influenza, or LPAI) caused mild flu in three children in Hong Kong: two in 1999 and in one child in mid-December 2003.
- H7N7 (HPAI) in the the Netherlands in February 2003 infected poultry, pigs, and people. By April the virus spread to nearly 800 poultry farms and ultimately resulted in the culling of almost 30 million chickens. An experienced veterinarian who'd visited one of the infected farms died from acute respiratory distress syndrome (ARD), a common complication of severe influenza. Eighty other poultry workers and their families developed mild flu, and were given Tamiflu. Of those eighty-eight cases, three were suspected to be person-to-person transmission (from the poultry workers to family members). There have been no other H7N7 cases in people since then.

  The total economic loss was estimated to be 700 million euros. From one outbreak, in one small country.
- H7N3 (HPAI) in British Columbia, Canada, in 2004 caused two cases of mild flu in two poultry workers. About 17 million chickens were slaughtered in an effort to stamp out any spread of the virus.

OTHER OUTBREAKS OF OTHER BIRD FLU VIRUSES IN THE UNITED STATES

The U.S. Department of Agriculture tracks and reports the various outbreaks of bird flu in this country. Most are not contagious, as only a scant few people have gotten sick. No one in America has died from contracting any of these viruses.

There have been three major outbreaks of High Pathogenic Avian Influenza (HPAI) in the United States—in 1924, 1983, and 2004.

The 1983 outbreak led to the destruction of 17 million birds in Pennsylvania and Virginia before that virus was finally contained and eradicated. No people were infected.

- H7N2 (HPAI) in 2002 and 2003 infected one poultry worker in Virginia and one patient in New York. Both recovered.
- H5N2 (HPAI) in 2004 in Texas and Pennsylvania. This outbreak was quickly found and eradicated after being confined to one flock of 6,600 birds. Still, hundreds of thousands of chickens were destroyed. This was bad news (and not just for the chickens) as this was the first major outbreak of an HPAI in America in over twenty years.
- H7N2 in 2004 in birds in Delaware and New Jersey. A month later, it appeared in birds in Maryland, and was likely the same strain.

Then—duck, duck, goose—it will infect poultry.

One of the reasons H5N1 can spread with such determined efficiency in poultry is a direct result of their environment. Much of the poultry on family farms in China is given "free range" to peck around the yard (and often all over the house itself). In America, the vast majority of chickens are hatched, reared, and slaughtered in enormous "factories." Unlike the happy little cluckers beloved of children in their storybooks and cartoons, few chickens live on family farms here anymore.

The Humane Society of the United States is not very sanguine about the prospects of controlling H5N1, given the conditions suffered by most commercially bred poultry in the United States (and abroad). Warehoused in incredibly cramped and disgustingly unsanitary conditions, breathing in and sleeping in their own waste, commercially raised chickens have a short and miserable life. They never see the light of day.

"There's been an exponential increase in High Pathogenic Avian Influenza outbreaks in the last twenty years. We believe that the killer H5N1 mutant is a virus of our own hatching," Michael Greger, M.D., director of public health and animal agriculture in the farm animal section of the Humane Society, told me. "Cramming tens of thousands of chickens bred to be almost genetically identical into filthy sheds to stand and lay beak-to-beak in their own feces is a recipe for increasing the virulence and transmission of this virus. It's an ideal breeding ground not just for suffering chickens but also for viral super-strains.

"Until we rethink and educate ourselves about factory-raised chickens, there will be no incentive to change the manner in which these chickens are reared," he adds. "The possibility of a pandemic is a very high price to pay for cheap food."

Imported Birds

I spoke to Dr. Teresa Telecky, former director of the Wildlife Trade Program at the Humane Society International and currently a consultant there, and she provided an illuminating look at how the trade in wild birds could also be a contributing factor to the spread of H5N1.

"Every year, 400,000 live exotic birds are legally imported into the United States for the pet trade," she told me. In addition, live birds reared for human consumption are sold at markets in San Francisco, Los Angeles, and New York. In 2004, birds from four live animal markets in New Jersey were found to carry a strain of avian influenza (not H5N1).

According to the USDA, more than 20 million birds of various species pass through as many as 150 known storefront slaughter facilities in the northeast metropolitan areas alone each year. Are these operations subject to USDA food safety regulations? No, they're not. Operations that process fewer than 20,000 birds per year are exempt. Translation: sick birds can get into the food chain. Or they can expose anyone who's worked with them or been near them to a bird virus.

Equally scary is the sheer number of illegally imported wild birds that enter our country every year. In other words, they're smuggled. Under coats, in luggage, on ships, in the trunks of cars driven over the border. They're subject to no regulation or oversight whatsoever. They could be sick with any number of diseases and we'd have no way of knowing who brought them in or where they were sold. (Dr. Telecky estimates that number to be at least 100,000 each year.)

China as well as countries in the European Union have banned any trade in wild birds, since they can't guarantee that these birds haven't come from areas infected with bird flu. But the smugglers could care less. They don't care about birds, or bird flu. They'd only care if their birds all died and they couldn't make a profit selling them to their regular customers.

"We can't control the illegally imported bird trade, but we can control the *legally* imported birds. They're all subject to quarantine when they come to the States," Dr. Telecky explains. "But each time birds are transported, there are many sites where they're handled—at facilities in different airports, in different countries—*prior* to quarantine. So everyone who's handling those birds can become infected.

"Viruses in birds are often asymptomatic, and blood tests are the only way to find out which one might be present. It can take days for symptoms to develop. That's why we're so worried about these handlers."

Every time wild exotic birds come into contact with people—not just the handlers, but those who buy them (that means you, bird owners!)— the potential exists for a preexisting bird virus to mix with a preexisting human virus. That can be Ground Zero for a new, mutant, highly contagious, and lethal virus.

"Nobody who works in the industry wants birds to get sick and spread disease, of course," she adds. "The breeders are very worried about the flu. The importers, on the other hand, could care less. If bird imports are banned, they'll simply switch to reptiles or amphibians.

"So we feel we have to take the most precautionary approach, and ban all trade in birds at the moment. Birds bred and reared in other countries can carry all sorts of disease, and spread it around the world.

"We also recommend that no one consider purchasing any wild birds now as pets."

(For more information about precautions around pet birds, see page 172.)

Cockfighting

Yes, you read it right. Cockfighting could be a contender in the spread of bird flu.

Cockfighting is illegal in forty-eight states and the District of Columbia; it's still legal in Louisiana and New Mexico. As all interstate transportation or export of birds for fighting purposes is prohibited by the federal Animal Welfare Act, cockfighting aficionados have been forced to go underground in this country. They're not about to stop any time soon on basic humanitarian grounds as they simply earn far too much money from the spectators who flock (sorry!) to the fights.

They flock to fights not just to watch roosters tear each other to shreds in despicably gory and painful bouts—they come to gamble. And there's an awful lot of money to be made during cockfighting "derbies." A recent raid by the FBI in Tennessee found takings of over a cool million bucks—from one night's fighting alone.

With that kind of money exchanging hands, cockfighting isn't going anywhere in hurry. Even though it's a felony to have fights or to possess any cocks for fighting in thirty states and the District of Columbia. And forty states and the District of Columbia prohibit being a spectator at cockfights. In the other states, fight promoters will only get a slap on the wrist and a small fine, and then get right back to it.

And if cockfighting is a hugely profitable underground spectator sport in America, it's positively massive in Asia. Bouts are even televised in Thailand and the Philippines.

Which brings us back to bird flu.

And some very, very worrisome information.

In 2002, there was an outbreak of Exotic Newcastle Disease (END), a deadly respiratory disease that can infect all bird species. After originating in California, it spread to Arizona, Nevada, New Mexico, and Texas. Over four million birds were ordered destroyed, and it cost the government more than $200 million on containment and compensation.

Needless to say, this was a health disaster for the affected poultry, and an economic disaster for poultry farmers.

The link from END to bird flu is cockfighting.

In a letter he wrote to the California State Senate in July, 2003, Dr. Richard Breitmeyer, California's state veterinarian, stated, "Game fowl and their owners have played a major role in the dissemination of the END virus due to their high mobility related to meetings, training, breeding, and fighting activities on a regular basis."

Because cockfighting has basically gone underground, it's as unregulated as the bird-smuggling trade. Tens of thousands of fighting cocks move all around the United States on a daily basis. If they catch any kind of avian disease, they can easily spread it, wherever they go.

As if that isn't horrific enough, during a fight, the cocks can't escape, regardless of how exhausted or injured they might be. They sustain severe injuries since their legs are fitted with razor-sharp steel blades or with gaffs, which are three inches long and look like curved ice picks. The blades and gaffs are designed solely to puncture and mutilate other cocks. Winner or loser, all the cocks suffer terribly. The sport is positively barbaric.

Here's the rub: Where there are injured cocks, there are cock handlers who get covered in their blood and other bodily fluids. (At some derbies, there are over five hundred roosters participating. Half are killed. The other half are injured, often severely. Multiply this figure by the sheer number of regularly scheduled, illegal, impossible-to-track cockfighting bouts, and you've got a lot of bloody, gory roosters.) Now, bird flu is not transmissible via tainted blood, as the AIDS virus is. But a bird that's been cut to shreds will have blood in its lungs. H5N1 being a respiratory virus, it thrives in the lungs and in certain bodily fluids, namely rooster mucus.

The most grotesque part: "There's a lot of hands-on interaction between the handlers and the roosters in all cockfights," John Goodwin, deputy manager for animal fighting issues at the Humane Society, told me. "When an injured cock is spitting up blood, its handler will put his mouth over the cock's beak to suction out the blood.

"We've been told that at least several of those killed by bird flu in Thailand were directly involved in cockfighting."

And if half the roosters in a cockfight are killed and the other half injured, those that survive are going to need a lot of handling—by people—to help them recuperate from their injuries. Naturally, they'll be drooling and dripping bodily fluids all over the place.

Goodwin and his colleagues know that they haven't got a chance at shutting down cockfighting abroad, but they're working hard to stiffen the fines with the ultimate goal of eradicating it completely in America.

"The problem is, bird flu is still seen as a joke among those in the cockfighting community in the United States. They're not taking the possible risks seriously," Goodwin told me. "Even in Thailand, there's still tremendous ignorance about how bird flu can be transmitted from infected roosters."

Astonishingly, thousands of owners of the fifteen million fighting cocks in Thailand held a rally in Suphanburi province on November 24, 2005, demanding that their birds be vaccinated. Naturally, they're the last people who'd demand a ban on their livelihood. Instead of putting an end to the fighting, they want the vaccines to do their dirty work for them.

"After the bird flu killed those men, the Thai government enacted a temporary ban on all blood sport. But we know it's being defied all the time," Goodwin adds. "At one checkpoint, a rooster fell out of one man's backpack, right at the policeman's feet. I think it's insane to defy the law, given what the consequences could be."

Pretty sickening, I'd say. And a pretty stupid way to die. Or set a pandemic in motion. (The ban on cockfighting in Thailand was scheduled to be lifted in January 2006.)

All for the chance to gamble on an inhumane "sport."

Patient Zero

Once those of us working in the infectious disease community were able to track the origins of the AIDS virus, we were able to identify a sexually active man from Montreal, who moved to New York. We called him Patient Zero.

We were able to track the Patient Zero carrier of West Nile virus in 1999. He flew into New York from Israel.

We were also able to track one Patient Zero who carried the SARS virus out of China, where it took only a month to spread to Vietnam, Singapore, and Canada, before moving into nearly thirty countries on six continents. Another Patient Zero from Hong Kong brought the SARS virus to Toronto, Canada, where she infected her son. Hundreds of other Canadians got sick and several dozen died.

Will there be a bird flu Patient Zero? Perhaps a poultry worker from China, who comes to America to visit his relatives, and doesn't know he's been infected. He's still asymptomatic. He sneezes all over passengers on the several planes he takes on his journey. He coughs all over people waiting for their luggage in the airport. He blows his nose in crowded restaurants. And when he suddenly develops a high fever and can barely move, he's rushed to a hospital, where he coughs and sneezes on all the patients waiting to be triaged. The language barrier prevents him from being questioned and immediately put into quarantine.

This is just one of countless scary scenarios.

Since all the other factors I talked about in chapter 1 have to be in place, this hypothetical Patient Zero can't really cause a pandemic all on his own. The virus he's carrying will have to have undergone the mutation it needs so it can spread efficiently from person to person. But when that mutation happens, a lot of people will be getting very sick.

Bottom line: We just don't know yet precisely how H5N1 will arrive.

But when it does, we'll want it gone.

Chapter 5.

BETTING *on* BIRD FLU— *the* REAL RISKS

This virus is very treacherous. While we cannot predict when or if the H5N1 virus might spark a pandemic, we cannot ignore the warning signs. We must act now if we are to have the maximum possible opportunity to contain a pandemic.

—*Dr. Margaret Chan, representative of the World Health Organization's Director-General for Pandemic Influenza*

We've been lucky so far.

Despite tens of millions of infected birds, the H5N1 bird flu has *not* shown the propensity to infect a lot of people—despite ample opportunity to do so.

If it did, we'd have a global pandemic already.

Why, then, does there seem to be a crisis in the making?

Why has the World Health Organization (WHO), the United Nations' agency for health and the one that's responsible for monitoring disease outbreaks around the globe, been sounding the alarm for nearly two years?

THE REAL RISK OF BIRD FLU

First of all, what's so different about this outbreak of H5N1?

Most of the countries currently fighting off H5N1 have never had to deal with an outbreak of High Pathogenic Avian Influenza (HPAI).

Ever.

This scope and size of this outbreak in birds is unprecedented.

The WHO has stated that "the current outbreaks of High Pathogenic Avian Influenza are the largest and most severe on record. Never before in the history of this disease have so many countries been simultaneously affected, resulting in the loss of so many birds."

Compared to the initial outbreak in 1997, and the subsequent outbreak in 2004, the current H5N1 strain is more lethal then ever. It mutates very rapidly. It kills more quickly. It kills more different species more quickly. (Animals such as mice and ferrets have been intentionally infected in laboratories in order to test their response to H5N1, and they got extremely sick, extremely fast.) A virus that had previously lived harmlessly in wild fowl intestines has mutated into something that was able to kill them.

In November 2005, the journal *Respiratory Research* reported a study conducted by researchers at the University of Hong Kong who studied the inflammatory response induced by H5N1 in laboratory-cultured human lung cells. They looked at levels of pro-inflammatory proteins called cytokines and chemokines.

The lung cells infected with the normal, seasonal flu virus had levels of the IL-10 chemokine at 200 picograms/milliliter. Those lung cells infected with H5N1 showed the IL-10 chemokine at nearly 2,000 picograms. That's nearly ten times more chemokine—which means that the immune system's inflammatory response to this virus is extremely aggressive.

Other studies had already shown that H5N1 increases the production of pro-inflammatory proteins in other cells. And inflammation—when organs and tissues are overwhelmed with blood and fluids in the body's attempt to fight off an infection—is what kills people with the flu.

Why is this happening now?

Everyone who lives through troubled times asks, why now? When it comes to viral activity, we can expect structural changes—mutation, reassortment, and recombination—to occur as days, months, even years go by. That's simply what viruses do. Through sheer bad luck, as well as other factors, this particular H5N1 virus is strengthening in power right now and killing millions of birds.

There have to be factors, some of which we understand and some of which we don't, which cause any kind of undulation in any virus's structure. If we could precisely pinpoint these factors, we might be able to predict pandemics with a higher degree of accuracy. But as we don't yet know what the factors are, we can only piece them together *as* they unfold, rather than *prior* to their unfolding.

Certainly, according the experts I've spoken to at the Humane Society, current practices of animal husbandry—in overcrowded, dank, and dismal chicken factories in particular—may very likely be at least partially responsible for the spread of the bird flu. As American soldiers were crammed into cramped and dirty barracks prior to being shipped off to war in 1918, giving the virus an unusually ample opportunity to spread, so are chickens crammed into festering, shockingly unhygienic sheds in 2006.

After all, this strain of the virus originated in countries where there are scant, if any, controls over how animals are raised. Nor is there a rapid system of informing citizens in isolated, nonelectrified rural communities, who may be dependent on their personal flocks for survival, about the dangers these chickens and ducks might be posing to others in the flock—as well as to their owners.

What is our real risk of a pandemic developing?

We already know that pandemics occur with regular ferocity. Some are mild, relatively speaking. Others are staggeringly lethal.

Over the last 160 years, there have been five pandemics: 1847–1848, 1889–1890, 1918–1919, 1957–1958, and 1967–1968.

"The world recognizes that this is a major public health challenge," claimed Dr. Lee Jong-wook, Director-General of the WHO, at a global meeting on November 9, 2005. "WHO is ready to focus its resources to reduce the risk of a human pandemic. We have plans on paper, but we must now test them. Once a pandemic virus appears, it will be too late."

That's not exactly reassuring.

The CDC and the U.S. Department of Agriculture aren't exactly resting idly, either. They're worried. And they should be.

They're worried due to the simple, ineluctable fact I talked about in chapter 2.

Viruses replicate. That's their sole function.

And when they replicate, they mutate.

The more these viruses have an opportunity to mutate, the higher the likelihood that they'll mutate into a new and more virulent version—at least from the virus's machinelike point of view. Remember, viruses aren't alive. They can't think, or plot, or say to themselves, let's get global with it and cause a pandemic. They just keep invading cells and replicating and doing what viruses have always done for billions of years.

For that reason, viruses that don't cause so much as a sneeze (Low Pathogenic Avian Influenza—LPAI) in birds (much less people) can transform themselves into mutant killers (High Pathogenic Avian Influenza—HPAI).

According to Dr. Ron DeHaven of the Animal and Plant Health Inspection Service (APHIS) division of the U.S. Department of Agriculture: "Research has shown that certain avian influenza virus strains, initially of low pathogenicity, can mutate—within six to nine months— into a highly pathogenic strain if allowed to circulate in poultry populations."

Six to nine months! No way is that enough time to develop and administer a brand-new vaccine, for either birds or people. That's why it's so crucial to contain the virus (by killing infected flocks) before it has a chance to spread, recombine through reassortment, and morph into a monster.

Since you read in the previous chapter about how the already highly pathogenic H5N1 is on the move—giving it more opportunity to infect new hosts—the possibility of it mutating from a virus transmitted from bird to bird into one transmitted from person to person is very real.

Now remember what I talked about in chapter 1: The stage is set for pandemics when four conditions have been met:

1. A virus pathogenic for humans establishes a global presence in an animal reservoir
2. There must be a new flu virus subtype to which the population is immunologically naïve (in other words, have no immunity)
3. The new virus infects people, and they get seriously ill
4. The virus is easily spread from person to person

Unfortunately, H5N1 has now fulfilled three of the four steps.

1. A virus pathogenic for humans establishes a global presence in an animal reservoir
2. It is a new virus in people (although it's not a new virus in birds)
3. It's infected 142 people, with a 50 percent mortality rate.

If H5N1 mutates into an easily transmissible virus any time soon, no person on this planet will have any natural immunity to it.

As I've said, H5N1 has not yet shown any propensity to make that crucial jump from bird-to-human to human-to-human. If it does, and if we do have a pandemic with a death rate similar to the 1918 Spanish Flu's death rate, the final global toll could be anywhere from 175 to 350 million dead.

Which means the real risk is pretty bad, right?

Let's just say it's serious. Not enough to make you want to run off and buy a case of surgical masks and plan to move off the electrical grid and live off the land. But serious enough to stay informed and follow developments as they unfold.

The WHO has H5N1 graded as a Stage 3 pandemic alert, with no or very limited human-to-human transmission. As long as H5N1 continues to spread and infect few new victims, the alert will remain at Stage 3.

It will take years to eradicate H5N1 from Asia (if indeed that can be done). In November 2005, China announced an audacious plan to vaccinate all 14 billion birds in that country. Yes, *14 billion!* Since two shots are needed for every bird, that's *28 billion* shots, each one administered by hand. It's an ambitious and overdue idea, and is certainly to be applauded, but logistically, how long do you think it will take to jab 14 billion squawking animals? Who'll be trained to do the (unpleasant) job? Given how many chickens live on family farms (and can be hidden), how feasible is this plan? And what if the virus morphs into something against which the vaccine turns out to be useless? (I'll talk more about vaccines in chapter 7.)

In addition, infected birds are appearing in countries thousands of miles from the Asian countries where the virus first appeared. And as you know by now, the longer any virus sticks around, and the more places it sticks around in, the higher the risk that it will infect people.

Then, the more those people get sick, the more the virus has a chance to fine-tune and improve its transmissibility to other people, allowing it to make that fatal jump that will transform its from a bird-to-person virus and into a person-to-person virus.

What is particularly worrisome is that H5N1 is so virulent. It's virulent in the same way that the 1918 Spanish Flu was. Remember that the plain, old, regular flu is a respiratory virus that first destroys the epithelial cells that guard against invading germs in your upper respiratory tract. If those cells are destroyed, it's much easier to get sick with pneumonia in the lungs, often caused by a secondary, bacterial infection. This explains why the very young and the very old, as well as the immuno-compromised, are most likely to die from the flu each year.

As I said in chapter 1, the Spanish Flu upended that scenario. It was able to burrow so deep inside the lungs, provoking an overwhelming immune response from the body desperate to get rid of it. As their lungs quickly filled with fluid and blood, victims literally drowned. And those who were most able to mount this attack on the virus were those with the strongest, most efficient immune systems—namely, young and healthy adults. That's why so many people between the ages of twenty and forty died so quickly and so terribly.

If the current H5N1 virus remains able to get deep inside the lungs, as it seems to be doing right now, then it, too, could kill those who seem most unlikely to die from it: the young and healthy.

It's simply too soon to know if this possibility will become reality.

At www.intrade.com you can place a bet on when bird flu will reach the United States. Right now, the betting points to a 50 percent chance the bird flu will arrive here in early 2006. What's worrisome is that these markets have been surprisingly accurate.

Let's hope that this time, they're wrong.

Does this mean I can stop worrying?

A healthy dollop of realism is what's needed.

Coupled with common sense. Hope for the best; prepare for the worst. That means you should get your house in order. But, of course, every adult in this country ought to have his or her house in order anyway, if only to be ready for any kind of natural or man-made disasters. Certainly what happened in the aftermath of the horrific hurricane season of 2005 should be enough to convince all of us to stock up on supplies such as food, water, and medications, have a first-aid kit, a will, adequate insurance, a family emergency meeting plan, and more. (See chapter 9 for more about preparation for a possible pandemic.)

And let's talk for a minute about how few cases there have been so far.

Right now, the world's population is about 6.6 billion. As of the end of 2005, there have been 142 cases of the bird flu in people in five different countries (Vietnam, Thailand, Indonesia, Cambodia, and China). Of these 142, 74 have died. This is a case-mortality rate of more than 50 percent. Not good for those who've gotten infected. Not good at all.

We don't know how many of the 6.6 billion humans on the planet have been infected; some may be asymptomatic or mildly ill. But those who have become ill with H5N1 represent such a relatively minute number of people that they aren't even a blip on the global population radar. Naturally, it goes without saying that this is no consolation to the families and loved ones of those who've died.

For those working on the front lines to prevent a pandemic, though, it is heartening news. The longer H5N1 takes to mutate into a potentially pandemic-inducing virus, the longer we have to try to contain it and fight it. To develop and administer new vaccines. To develop and provide potent anti-viral medications. To get information out there so no one panics.

In fact, the Infectious Disease Society of America (IDSA), recently put together a subcommittee to track and study H5N1, and they've made some broad recommendations about the sort of the direction they think we should be moving in. These recommendations aren't precise, or specific, because the IDSA's stance is that of long-range planning, over the next five years, which, theoretically, means that many in the infectious disease community believe we may have that amount of time.

But practically every day, it seems there's another scare story in the media. Who am I to believe?

When the Spanish Flu pandemic took off with lethal speed in the fall of 1918, public health officials and the media made some terrible decisions that may have costs tens of thousands of citizens their lives. "Don't Get Scared" appeared in newspapers in nearly every city in this country. The headline should have blared: "Stay Home."

John Robertson, then the public health commissioner in Chicago, arrogantly stated, "It is our duty to keep people from fear. Worry kills more people than the epidemic."

With that flu, however, he was wrong. *Dead* wrong.

In retrospect, of course, it's easy to point a condemning finger. Our country was at war, and people were already on edge. Such a virulent pandemic had never touched so many people at the same time; certainly, no one ever expected that the highest death toll would occur in young, healthy adults. But those who watched their neighbors succumb knew what was going on. Where was the leadership in our country?

Now, thankfully, we have the opposite—not a paltry dribble of misinformation meant to reassure people while doing nothing of the sort, but accurate and updated information posted on reputable websites belonging to the CDC and WHO, among others. The infectious disease community, the CDC, and WHO have been quietly tracking and evaluating H5N1 since it appeared in Hong Kong in 1997. When it returned with a vengeance in 2003, we began to be increasingly vigilant—and concerned.

Articles in the press began to appear when there were fatalities in people, but, frankly, a few dozen rural farmers dying in rural Vietnam wasn't exactly of earth-shattering importance to Americans going about their busy, daily lives. Sounds harsh, but it's true. Frankly, millions of people have died in the Sudan of late; millions more are infected and dying from AIDS-related illness in poor Third World countries, but until tragic situations physically touch us, here at home, we're basically a pretty complacent and insulated society.

The media began to wake up to the H5N1 situation as more deaths were reported, in different countries. Then, Hurricane Katrina made a direct hit on the Louisiana coast. The ensuing tragedy was a terrifying jolt of in-our-face reality about our country's terrifying inability to mount a swift response to a long-expected and devastating natural disaster.

What seemed to be the tipping point for the American media with the current bird flu situation was when migratory birds brought the virus to Europe. H5N1 was discovered in Turkey, Romania, Croatia, and Greece in the fall of 2005. Since then, it's been suspected in Canada.

Those countries are a lot closer to us than Vietnam or Indonesia.

As winter drew near, those birds gotta keep flying.

And when President Bush unveiled a $7.1 billion plan (of which only $3.8 billion was approved by Congress in December 2005) to deal with the threat of an H5N1 pandemic on November 1, 2005, it was official. Bird flu was for real. It was acknowledged by the White House as a serious threat not just to America but to the world.

Reporters went into overdrive. "Are We Ready?" blared the headlines.

Avian influenza is not a story that's going to go away anytime soon. For one thing, pandemics do occur, one is statistically overdue, and H5N1 has an extremely high potential for mutation. This is not hype. It's reality.

As H5N1 spreads into more flocks of birds and into people, and mutations occur, it will continue to be relevant and newsworthy. The numbers are staggering: 14 *billion* birds in China to get vaccines; hundreds of *billions* of dollars in potential economic losses; *billions* of people who may become infected; tens of *millions* who may die. This is not hype, either.

In essence, we are eyewitnesses to a potential global catastrophe, watching and waiting as it unfolds before our eyes.

I should think that anyone reading this book already knows the dif- ference between reality and hype—and that hype sells. It sells newspa- pers and magazines, and it entices people to watch TV so they can be bombarded by more things for sale. That's the way the world works in a media-and-advertising-driven world. The more sensational, the more likely we are to read all about it, or stay glued to the screen. It's just hu- man nature.

Hype can be dangerous, though. Continual warnings about potential catastrophes are like the proverbial chicken running around screaming, "The sky is falling! The sky is falling!" (Particularly apt with this virus, don't you think?) When the sky doesn't fall, people tune out. They be- come complacent. They're sure nothing is going to happen in their area, or if it did, it wouldn't happen to them.

Residents of New Orleans found out just how dangerous hype and unheeded warnings can be, sadly enough. To be fair, many who were told to evacuate had no means of transportation to do so. But some who did had already evacuated during previous hurricane warnings, and then those storms veered away at the last moment, and nothing much hap- pened save a few felled trees. These people weren't about to be inconve- nienced again—with tragic results.

Actually, we've already lived through two other media frenzies about two different viruses in recent years.

For the first, we have to go back three decades, to the year of the Bi- centennial, 1976, when swine flu caused a national crisis. Back then, Pres- ident Gerald Ford famously rolled up his sleeve and got his swine flu shot without a wince, then watched as public confidence (and his reelection prospects) sank more quickly that you could say Tricky Dickie.

For the second, we don't have to go back three decades. We only have to go back three years. Remember when SARS was the Scare du Jour? SARS also was a virus that appeared out of nowhere, and went from zero to sixty seemingly overnight. The media went berserk. Travelers strapped on face masks and peered anxiously over them in airports. The world was on edge. People were beginning to panic.

Until the virus disappeared as quickly as it appeared.

The swine flu scare of 1976 is now not much more than a footnote to all the factors contributing to a president's demise, but at the time—

according to the media, at least—it was the Big One. As for SARS, well, do you still remember any details about it? Although it appeared barely three years ago, unless you traveled to or from China during the height of the epidemic, you probably don't. Other, more recent and catastrophic disasters have, unfortunately, displaced it from the public consciousness. And since SARS doesn't seem to be a threat anymore, why bother thinking about it—right?

So allow me to refresh your memory, as I think it's extremely useful to go back to these two previous scares and see how the media responded to what seemed to be new threats at the time.

ABOUT SWINE FLU

When an eighteen-year-old private doing his basic training at Fort Dix, New Jersey, came down with the flu on February 4, 1976, no one thought much about it. That winter was particularly brutal, and lots of other soldiers had come down with nasty bouts of the flu, too. But they didn't die from it.

This private did.

This was a bad shock. The young man had been glowing with health only a few days before. All the soldiers on the base were young, vibrant men in robust physical shape. And scientists at the CDC were even more shocked when a swab taken from the dead private tested positive for swine flu. By then, four other soldiers lay sick with the same virus.

Swine flu has been around for eons, as has bird flu. But it wasn't normally a virus that was transmitted from pigs to people, or if it was, it wasn't a killer. This swine virus, coupled with the fact that a healthy young soldier had died so quickly from it, brought back very unpleasant memories and fears. Was this virus similar to the bird virus that had caused the 1918 pandemic? Was it a recurrence, or just a fluke?

President Ford and the epidemiologists at the CDC had a quandary on their hands. If a swine flu epidemic took flight and there were no vaccines, millions might die. (Anti-viral drugs hadn't been invented yet.) But if the CDC insisted that vaccines were necessary, it would cost a bundle to develop, manufacture, and distribute them, based only on the death of one soldier in New Jersey and the hypothetical possibility that an epidemic *might* happen.

It was a tough call, and President Ford decided to err on the side of caution. He asked Congress to appropriate $135 million. It was a tough battle, as drug manufacturers did not want to assume any liability from potential side effects of the vaccine. Many scientists claimed that the sole death was not an indication of an epidemic in the making. By August, the National Influenza Immunization Program (NIIP) was stalled in Congress.

Now, here's where this tale gets a little crazy.

When the swine flu scare started, the media was calling for immediate action. As in: Get those vaccines in our arms, right this minute. Then, as no one else seemed to be getting sick with swine flu, the tide turned. Suddenly, there was an outbreak of a particularly lethal strain of pneumonia at the 1976 Pennsylvania State Convention of the American Legion. Of the 182 legionnaires who got sick, 29 of them died.

At the time, no one knew that what would eventually be called Legionnaire's Disease was neither the flu nor caused by a virus. But the media decided, with not a whole lot of evidence to do so, that this outbreak of pneumonia had to be related to swine flu, so let's get those shots back on track.

Amazingly, by October 1, the vaccines were good to go. Thousands lined up and dutifully stuck out their arms. Until, on October 12, three elderly people near Pittsburgh collapsed from heart attacks at the vaccination station and died hours after being inoculated. The entire vaccination program was immediately suspended in Pennsylvania.

The media, which only two months before had been fairly screaming for vaccines, now did an abrupt about-face, exaggerating the risks of complications from the shots. Nine other states shut down their vaccination programs, until the CDC released proof that the heart attack victims had not died from the shots themselves.

That did little to dampen public concern—and by December, the public had a right to be concerned. Guillain-Barré syndrome, a rare neurological disease that can cause paralysis and death, was suddenly appearing in alarmingly high numbers, given its rarity. For those who were susceptible, the vaccine may have somehow triggered a detrimental immune response. The only causative link appeared to be the swine flu shot.

With dozens of families screaming for (and eventually receiving) recompense in blaring headlines, and with public confidence in government-sanctioned preventative health measures at a new low, the NIIP program was suspended. Dr. David Senser, the then head of the Centers for Disease Control, was fired as a scapegoat for this difficult chapter in the history of our nation's public health system. Over 40 million people had gotten flu shots for a nonexistent flu epidemic. Later research on that particular strain of flu showed that even had it spread, it would not have been anywhere as devastating as the 1918 strain.

Some good did come from this fiasco (especially if you were a fan of Jimmy Carter, who won the presidency in 1976). Vaccine manufacturers proved that they were able to create and produce tens of millions of doses in an exceedingly short time. They were able to use state-of-the-art technology to create a new formulation—what's called an attenuated vaccine—which utilized whole virus that had been chemically weakened, instead of purified split virus.

The truth be told, if the swine flu epidemic had ever materialized into a pandemic, the relatively small number of cases of Guillain-Barré syndrome would have be considered acceptable balanced against the hundreds of thousands that might have been saved.

Where the media's concerned, though, fingers can still be pointed. Much of the reporting at the time was designed not to inform, but to sensationalize and scare. The fickleness of the "We Don't Need the Shot–We Do Need the Shot–The Shot Kills–We Never Said You Should Get the Shot" reporting left the public uninformed about the real risks, and quite cynical about public health initiatives. This could prove to have devastating results today, should we have a real epidemic or pandemic on our hands.

When doomsday scenarios mercifully don't unfold in the way they're expected to, the media can turn around and shoot the messenger, without accepting any culpability for creating the doomsday scenarios in the first place. And all this happened long before the Internet was a gleam in a programmer's eye.

Given the "It's a Killer–It's Not a Killer" articles appearing now about the bird flu, I can't fault my patients who are seriously misinformed about what's going on. If (allegedly) reputable newspapers and networks can't present the news in a calm and thoroughly researched manner, how can the public know what to believe?

ABOUT SARS

SARS was a previously unknown virus that appeared with no warning in rural China in February of 2003. Called SARS, the acronym for Severe Acute Respiratory Syndrome, SARS turned out to be caused by a coronavirus originating in wild civet cats. These cats live in rural China, where they're eaten and considered a delicacy.

SARS was spread by close person-to-person contact (as is the seasonal flu), by the droplets produced during coughs and sneezes, or by touching or being in prolonged contact—closer than three feet—with an infected person. So you could catch it when sitting next to an infected person, but not by walking past him or her on the street or in an airport. It was highly contagious, especially among health care workers. And like the seasonal flu, there was a rapid onset, with high fever, headache, aches, chills, and coughing. Most of its victims developed pneumonia, too.

When an infected doctor carried the virus out of China, it spread to Vietnam and Singapore and Canada within a month. Before long, the SARS virus had spread to nearly thirty countries on six continents.

Once they realized that this was a new and potentially devastating virus, the WHO and CDC kicked into overdrive, testing specimens from SARS patients to isolate and study the virus. Modern medical technology led to the rapid identification of the previously unknown coronavirus. The CDC activated its Emergency Operations Center to provide round-the-clock coordination and response; deployed medical officers, epidemiologists, and other specialists to assist with on-site investigations around the world; and helped state and local health departments with their investigations of possible SARS cases in the United States. They alerted airlines and travelers to Asia about the risks. All travel to Asia fell by nearly half (and the travel industry still hasn't recovered).

Naturally, this was covered in breathless detail by the media.

One of the biggest problems with the SARS reporting was due to the habitual secrecy of the Chinese government. Although the virus had originated in southern China, officials there initially lied about it. They either hid or pooh-poohed its spread.

Meanwhile, 349 innocent Chinese died while the government stonewalled. It wasn't until SARS had spread into Hong Kong and then around the world that the Chinese officials finally conceded that they had a problem. Thousands had perhaps unnecessarily become infected as a result. (To save face, China ordered that two senior officials be fired and blamed for the fiasco.)

After the outbreak ended, the WHO reported that a total of 8,098 people had been infected worldwide, with 774 fatalities. That made the case-mortality rate 9.5 percent.

Americans were very lucky. Only eight people here came down with SARS, and all of them had traveled to other parts of the world already infected by SARS, which is where they caught it. No cases originated in this country, and its spread was entirely contained. Although there still is not treatment for SARS, understanding of the mechanism of the coronavirus and its spread, as well as the animal host where it initially incubated, has stemmed the tide of human cases—at least for the present.

Aside from the loss of life, the economic cost to the Asian-Pacific region was staggering—about $40 billion.

Looking back, we dodged an enormous bullet. SARS did not develop into a pandemic. It didn't even develop into an epidemic, it was a limited outbreak lasting about six months. Thank goodness for that.

And SARS certainly impacted our awareness of viruses and epidemics and global health. I know that the experience we had at work, when in 2003 a suspected SARS patient was admitted to the Tisch Center/New York University Medical Hospital Center (as related in chapter 6), had a dramatic effect on our subsequent training and preparation for future outbreaks of communicable diseases. Initially, our procedures for isolation and patient care were untested and somewhat rusty, but systems were quickly honed to try and deal with it. I think it's a fair assumption that most other hospitals in America have undergone the same sort of preparation and put these protocols into place.

In addition, I believe that the increased vigilance and surveillance put into place by China after it was internationally chastised for downplaying the initial SARS outbreaks has helped with the initial detection of bird flu. While they were looking for sick people, local Chinese health officials trying to figure out where SARS came from were also on the lookout for all kinds of sick birds and animals, and sampling tens of thousands of them.

Then, when SARS disappeared, a big sigh of relief was heaved by public health officials, people threw their unused face masks away, and the media moved on to the next Big One. The problem, though, is that many skeptics about H5N1 are quick to point to the SARS scare as a tempest in a teapot, blown way out of proportion, especially as there had been no cases of it originating in America.

Of course, it's easy to say that in retrospect.

These skeptics ought to stop gloating, frankly. Simple reason: The coronavirus that caused SARS in no way resembles the H5N1 virus in its structure. Nor is the SARS virus closely related to any other pathogen. In other words, it's not a virus that's been around for eons like influenza— and because it's so new, it was not well adapted to the human population. (This is the likely explanation for its sudden demise.) So no one should take the short duration of SARS as proof that H5N1 might have the same kind of natural history.

Isn't it good, though, that we can instantly go on the Internet and read all about H5N1?

The Internet is a fantastic resource, no doubt about it.

Within reason.

When the AIDS epidemic started in the early 1980s, I spent endless hours in the library, leafing through piles of papers and heavy indices and medical tomes, and ordering abstracts from the librarian. I wrote letters to colleagues asking advice. Call-waiting seemed like manna from heaven, as it enabled me to get through to my patients much more quickly. And the fax machine—what a miracle to be able to instantly send a document to a colleague abroad! Who would have thought a decade ago that I'd now be able to push a few buttons on my computer and have immediate access to a staggering amount of useful information?

That's the good news. So much of what's on the Internet is incredibly valuable and easy to understand. The CDC and WHO websites have daily updates about H5N1. They link to other websites worldwide, especially health departments in other countries, for more statistics and facts and stories than you'd ever need to know. News services such as the Associated Press and Reuters post articles from their global network of reporters and sources instantaneously, and English-language editions of newspapers in Asian countries can also be accessed. Breaking news can be read immediately.

The bad news, of course, is that so much of what's on the Internet is incredibly wrong and not easy to avoid. Especially about science. These are sources that cannot be trusted.

At last Google of "bird flu," there were 38 million links. ("Avian influenza," the more proper and less colloquial term, had only 5.7 million. To put this figure into perspective, on the other hand, George Bush had 116 million and Madonna 29.8 million.)

Many of the links are to fearmongers out to make a quick buck off people's fears. They're simply updated versions of the hucksters who capitalized on fears in 1918, too, by blanketing newspapers with their ads ("Influ-BALM Prevents Spanish Flu!"; "Keep Your Mouth Clean—Use SOZODONT!").

When you do a Google search on bird flu, the ads appear on the right of your screen. "Lightning Air Purifier! Kills Bird Flu!" reads one. (Never mind that the virus isn't alive, so you can't kill it.) "Immune Defense Against the Flu!" "Bird Flu Protection!" "Prepare for Avian Bird Flu!" "Free Survival Tips!" "Join the Bird Flu Discussion! Gift Certificates for the Holidays!" "Flu Buster Might Be the Answer!"

Well, actually, no, it might not.

There is a simple way to avoid falling victim to hucksters. Stick to the facts. The CDC, WHO, and other reputable sites do not promote fearmongering. (See the Online Resources section on page 181 for links to useful sites.) They do not endorse or sell products. They do not recommend untested herbal formulas. They simply present information as it unfolds.

And then there are the bloggers.

If you like to read blogs, feel free, although when it comes to such an important topic, I'd advise an extremely healthy dose of skepticism. The mere fact of reading something on the Internet doesn't make it true— about the flu, or about anything else.

Some bloggers are actually quite knowledgeable about the flu. Others might be thought of as amusing if the talk about the flu is scaring you, and you need to find a spot of humor about it. A lot, however, are neither knowledgeable nor amusing. They post endless diatribes; they aren't written by experts; they aren't edited by anyone who may know more than they do; and they rarely check their sources. They answer to no one, so that any old crackpot theory that bloggers may have heard from someone who read about it somewhere or other—but is *absolutely* without question *certain* that it's true—suddenly becomes presented as "fact." Once it is, it can be thought of as such. That can be dangerously misleading. Especially when public health is at risk.

The sheer volume of attention that bird flu is getting—from accurate sources as well as from quacks—is scary in and of itself. Worse, it may be somewhat misleading for the average, concerned citizen who might understandably have trouble sifting through what's important and what's hustle and hype. A colleague's wife recently remarked to me that she had stopped reading anything that remotely mentioned bird flu. She had become so inundated with scare stories that she simply shut down into a firm state of denial—not a state I'd recommend, given the ever-shifting status of the H5N1 virus.

She did have a point, though. The surfeit of articles and television reports *can* be very confusing. I've had patients who've come in for their annual flu shots—educated, responsible patients who are dutiful about getting their vaccinations every year. They know enough about vaccines to understand that there are new strains of the seasonal flu each year, and that they need new immunity to them. But, with all this talk about bird flu swirling around, they'll still ask, "Does this protect me from the bird flu?"

Clearly, there is often a disconnect between what's in the news, and what people take away from those news reports. Too much information can mean that none of it is understood. Or understood properly.

For that reason, the Information Age is akin to a double-edge sword. It allows information to be immediately sent out, so that people can immediately respond in a crisis. If they're told to stay away from crowds during a flu outbreak, to not go to work or take their children to school, they'll do so. But too much information can paradoxically cause people to panic. If they develop any of what they fear are symptoms—because, after all, they read about them on the Internet—they might rush to a busy hospital where their risk factors might drastically increase, whereas if they'd only stayed home (and nursed what turned out to be a bad cold) they would not have put themselves in unnecessary danger.

And there's another point to consider: Science is not always accurate.

AT LEAST YOU CAN LAUGH

There's a joke making the rounds on the Internet:
"The Centers for Disease Control has released a list of symptoms of bird flu. If you experience any of the following, please seek medical treatment immediately:

1. High fever
2. Congestion
3. Nausea
4. Fatigue
5. Aching in the joints
6. An irresistible urge to shit on someone's windshield."

No, the CDC has not released such a list.
Then there's Cafépress.com, where just about anyone can hawk all sorts of ridiculous merchandise. There, you can buy tee shirts and magnets emblazoned with such phrases as "Cock-a-doodle flu," "Chicken's revenge—bird flu is coming," "If you're close enough to read this, you're close enough to catch my bird flu," "Prevent bird flu—choke your chicken," or "H5N1—One flu over the cuckoo's nest." One of the silliest has a picture of a bird over the phrase: "Did you just sneeze?"
Given the potential seriousness of a potential pandemic, laughing about it isn't such a bad idea. As long as you stay informed about it, too.

Doctors and scientists and researchers can be wrong. Hypotheses that were once put forward as irrefutable fact turned out to be incorrect years or even decades later.

That's why it's crucial to rely on reputable sources for your information about the bird flu.

Will H5N1 ever be completely eradicated?

Perhaps. It might disappear. It might mutate into something more benign. Or it might mutate into something so lethal, killing so many people that it runs out of hosts.

According to the WHO, the Asian countries struggling to contain the spread of H5N1 right now estimate that it will be several years before the virus can be controlled. As long as H5N1 continues to circulate in birds, so will the risk continue that it will transform itself into a virus that can spread among people with great speed.

Bottom line with pandemics: As much as we wish we could, we simply can't predict them with any accuracy. They're like trains rolling down the tracks. You can hear the rumbling but you don't always know which way it's going. It can be right on top of you—or it can pass you right by.

Chapter 6.

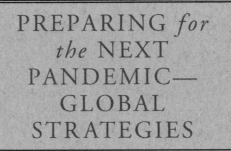

PREPARING *for* *the* NEXT PANDEMIC— GLOBAL STRATEGIES

The world recognizes that this is a major public health
challenge. WHO is ready to focus its resources to reduce the risk
of a human pandemic. We have plans on paper, but we
must now test them. Once a pandemic virus appears,
it will be too late.

—*Dr. Lee Jong-wook, Director-General of the*
World Health Organization (WHO)

When the Spanish Flu suddenly appeared in 1918, no one was prepared. Global communication was by telegraph wire; global travel was via steamship and train. Airplanes could only fly short distances; automobiles reached a top speed of about thirty miles an hour. Most people in rural areas were still entirely dependent on horses and wagons. Telephone service was hand-cranked, slow, and sporadic.

Even then, the H1N1 pandemic strain of the virus had encircled the world in less than six weeks.

Now, of course, we can hop on airplanes and encircle the world in only a day or two, spreading viruses before the flight attendants can say,

"Prepare for landing." We have the example of what went wrong when the Spanish Flu hit. Nevertheless, as we turn a wary eye on H5N1 and wonder if it will mutate into a lethal form transmissible to humans, at least we will be prepared for this to happen. It won't be an overwhelming surprise.

Even with all this warning, however, we still might be severely tested and found wanting—because despite all the blaring headlines and the hundreds of millions of dollars apportioned to vaccine development and stockpiling of anti-viral drugs, we are underprepared.

Pandemics hit everyone. They aren't localized as natural disasters like tsunamis and earthquakes are. From the remotest village on the Arctic Circle to the cultured lawns of Beverly Hills, from the pampas in Argentina to the forests of Siberia, from the rice paddies of Vietnam to the cafes in Vienna, we're all at risk.

To remove that fear from the public consciousness, and spurred on by the cogent urging of the WHO and other public health organizations, governments fearful of the enormous personal and economic toll should a pandemic hit are scrambling to put disaster plans in place *prior* to any outbreaks. Many of these programs are well intentioned and can work quite well on a local level. Others, especially in developing nations, suffer from lack of manpower, technological know-how, and financial resources despite the best intentions.

The possibility of a pandemic is a global problem. No one country can solve the problem; no one country can keep its borders safe.

Let's first take a look at what's being done in America. (I'll tackle personal preparation in chapter 9.)

THE PANDEMIC INFLUENZA PLAN FOR THE UNITED STATES

"To respond to a pandemic we must have emergency plans in place in all fifty states, in every local community," President George W. Bush has claimed. "We must ensure that all levels of government are ready to act to contain an outbreak."

The president and the Department of Health and Human Services (HHS), outlined their National Strategy for Pandemic Influenza with their Pandemic Influenza Plan on November 1, 2005. It had three distinct phases, each with different objectives:

Phase 1—Pre-pandemic
• Reduce opportunities for human infection
• Strengthen the early warning system through surveillance and detection

Phase 2—Emergence of a pandemic virus
• Contain or delay spread at the source

Phase 3—Pandemic declared and spreading internationally
• Reduce morbidity and mortality by limiting the spread of the outbreak and mitigating its health and economic impacts, and social disruption
• Conduct research to guide response measures

As stated in the National Strategy for Pandemic Influenza, it is intended to guide our preparedness and response to an influenza pandemic, with the intent of (1) stopping, slowing, or otherwise limiting the spread of a pandemic to the United States; (2) limiting the domestic spread of a pandemic, and mitigating disease, suffering, and death; and (3) sustaining infrastructure and mitigating impact to the economy and the functioning of society. The ultimate goal is for a state of national readiness and ability to quickly respond to a pandemic.

The White House is working in tandem with many other public health organizations, such as WHO, Food and Agriculture Organization (FAO), World Organization for Animal Health (OIE), the Asia-Pacific Economic Cooperation (APEC) forum, and other groups. It has delegated specific responsibilities to various federal departments: medical response (HHS and CDC), veterinary response (Department of Agriculture), international activities (Department of State), and domestic incident management and federal coordination (Department of Homeland Security—not that this is especially reassuring, given what happened after Hurricane Katrina).

The secretary of HHS, Michael Leavitt, further elaborated on specific planning procedures. The integral steps in this plan are:

- International surveillance
- Domestic surveillance
- Vaccine development
- Anti-viral medication
- Communication

I'll cover vaccine development in chapter 7 and anti-viral medications in chapter 8.

CURRENT BIRD FLU SURVEILLANCE STRATEGIES

As we are currently at the Stage 3 pandemic level, surveillance is critical.

Surveillance in the United States and other countries

At the recent twenty-fourth Conference for the Regional Commission for Asia, the Far East and Oceania division of the World Organization for Animal Health (OIE), the OIE's director general, Dr. Bernard Vallat, claimed, "I believe that there is still a window of opportunity for substantially reducing the risk of a human pandemic by minimizing the virus load in animals worldwide. Strengthening animal disease surveillance systems worldwide is essential for tracking the evolution of the pathogenic agent, which is crucial for the prevention of any future global crisis associated with emerging animal diseases potentially transmissible to humans."

Surveillance is not just about tracking outbreaks of avian influenza in the bird population. It's about increasing surveillance at the locations where people interact with birds—on farms, at live bird markets, at cockfights, at processing plants. It's also quite possible that the virus could be transported over vast distances in shipments of farm birds, or even vehicles traveling from virus-ridden areas. (Remember, the H5N1 can live in manure for a lot longer that you want to think about.)

To establish a viable, seamlessly functioning surveillance network, global cooperation is necessary. So are field laboratories to inspect samples, trained investigators, and rapid response teams.

And then there's the problem of paying for all of this. . . .

In the meantime, migratory birds are bringing H5N1 from Southeast Asia to north and central Asia and on to Europe. Cases may soon appear in Africa as flocks make their seasonal journeys from the northern European winter to warmer climates.

To prevent a pandemic, H5N1 outbreaks *must* be carefully monitored. It's imperative to know where the viral outbreaks are located, where they may be spreading, and if H5N1 is in the process of mutating. Since Type A influenza is such a common disease, confirmation of the H5N1 virus can, at the moment, only be performed by a WHO-associated lab. (During a pandemic, it would be assumed that H5N1 was the dominant strain, and testing would be moot.)

Satellite phones and e-mail have allowed the public health field workers (many of whom are with WHO) to transmit urgent messages from remote villages, which is a huge aid to surveillance. As soon as the field workers notice any new developments, they can report them.

Because H5N1 is so lethal, and kills flocks of birds—but *not*, as you know by now, all birds—in an extremely short amount of time, it's fair to assume that if it arrives in this country, we'll know it very quickly.

In October 2005, Agriculture Deputy Secretary Chuck Connor outlined the U.S. Department of Agriculture's efforts to protect us from H5N1. "Attacking the disease at its source overseas is a main focus for USDA," he said. "We also have strict importation restrictions to prevent the spread of the virus in our country and an elaborate surveillance system in place to monitor our bird populations."

This surveillance focuses on commercial poultry producers, where the Animal and Plant Health Inspection Service (APHIS) division of the USDA conducts over one million tests a year for different strains of avian influenza. In addition, the APHIS is working with state agricultural departments to increase surveillance at live bird markets around the country. They're also conducting a major outreach campaign called "Biosecurity for the Birds," in which they're educating both large poultry producers and farmers with small barnyard flocks about the dangers of bird flu, and encouraging them to immediately report sick birds.

Far more difficult in scope is surveillance of the wild bird population. Along with the USDA, surveillance is being supervised by the U.S. Geological Survey (experts about migratory birds and their movement), U.S.

Fish and Wildlife Service (which oversees refuges providing critical nesting, migration, and wintering habitat for waterfowl and other migratory birds as well as governing trade in wildlife species), and the National Park Service (which protects the health of its visitors).

Migratory birds in Alaska on the "Pacific Flyway" path have been sampled for the last several months, and more extensive surveillance is planned for the spring of 2006. It's believed that if H5N1 comes to America, it will most likely arrive from Asia via the Alaska route. Although there is no as-yet-documented evidence that stricken migratory birds survive long enough to carry H5N1 over long distances, the possibility can't be ruled out.

"Between Eastern Asia and the Pacific Northwest, there are numerous species that have regular paths of migration in which they nest in Alaska and on the North Slope and move southward away from winter conditions to over-winter in more temperate climates around the world," explained Dr. Richard Kearney, the Wildlife Program Coordinator at the U.S. Geological Survey. "We recognize the birds that are on the move now away from Alaska and North America are going to be over-wintering in areas in which we have observed outbreaks of H5N1. When these birds return in the spring, there's a possibility that a number may return with the virus."

As for surveillance in the human population, the CDC has been requesting that physicians send respiratory specimens from patients hospitalized with what is suspected to be Type A influenza, and who have recently traveled to countries with known outbreaks of H5N1, to their laboratory for further testing.

There is also extensive worldwide surveillance for new H5N1 outbreaks, overseen by WHO and OIE, who provide advice through a global network of experts, researchers, and laboratories, and send field workers to help with the watching. American experts would be sent to any areas abroad where any shifts in the virus, such as a new cluster of cases in people, seem to be unfolding.

In addition, the Convention on Migratory Species (CMS) has designed an international wildlife warning system to monitor migratory flocks for disease and to warn different countries about the potential for the arrival of H5N1 in seasonal movements of birds. It will take at least two years to have the monitoring system fully operational.

"Precise information on the places where migratory birds go, including their resting sites and final destinations, is currently scattered across a myriad of organizations, bodies, and groups," said Klaus Toepfer, executive director of the United Nations Environment Program (UNEP). "It is absolutely vital that this is brought together in a way that is useful to those dealing with the threat of this pandemic backed up by high quality, precision mapping."

While Asian countries that have experienced outbreaks are quietly trying to manage surveillance in the meantime, it isn't easy. After HHS chief Michael Leavitt returned from an Asian trip in the fall of 2005, he recounted a frightening tale: "I got up very early in the morning and went off to a wet market where I walked around large cages of turkeys and ducks and chickens and pigs all in the same area," he said. "And I hap-

GENETIC SURVEILLANCE

There are two projects underway which hold the promise of better understanding how human influenza is derived in the environment, and precisely which mutations herald the shift to more pathogenic strains. One of these is the Avian Influenza Genomic Project, a collaboration between the NIAID, The Institute for Genomic Research (TIGR), and Ohio State University. Entire genomes of thousands of strains of avian influenza recovered in the field from around the globe are being decoded and catalogued. Homology studies (testing the similarity of genomes from different sources) can help scientists understand the evolution, and the derivations of viral subtypes. From this work, the risks of shift from bird to human pathogen can be assessed, and the critical animal reservoirs can be identified and interrupted.

Another similar project is the Human Influenza Genome Project. Full genomes of over four hundred strains of influenza virus obtained from humans have been decoded, which have shown an incredible diversity in structure. These types of studies will ultimately further our understanding of how to keep one step ahead of a virus that is able to mutate, undergo reassortment, and move from host to host. Ultimately, it will be the science of influenza, that will help the government and public health policy makers determine where to make best use of their resources to control influenza disease.

pened to wake a woman up who was sleeping there who was a pig farmer." She had driven six hundred kilometers the night before with her pigs on the top of her bus—next to a group of chickens. "She was going to get up the next morning and sell them and return home. She lives in a very remote area where there isn't television or media."

As a result, she'd never even heard of bird flu. She had no idea that birds plus pigs plus people is an ideal mixing bowl for viral mutations.

"There are a wide variety of practices that we observe and a wide variety of surveillance available," Leavitt added. "The difficulty with the challenge that is faced by these governments that we want to be helpful to is that they're dealing with a situation where there isn't always a health care system where a person can report to. That's the difference in the variety of circumstances we're focused on helping."

So while surveillance strategies sound logical, they're still problematic not just in developing nations with little or no public health supervision—for two simple reasons.

It's impossible to have a comprehensive surveillance plan when millions and millions of migratory birds are constantly on the move . . . and when millions of innocent people are going about their lives without any realization that a pandemic might be brewing.

CURRENT RESPONSE STRATEGIES TO H5N1 OUTBREAKS

Each country has or is in the process of developing a plan/system to manage and try to curtail local outbreaks. This is especially critical in Asia.

If there is a bird flu pandemic, it won't hit only one fairly well-defined area, as do other natural disasters like hurricanes or tornados. It also wouldn't be constrained by geography, as are tsunamis or floods. It would spread extensively throughout the country in a very short span of time.

Nor would a pandemic quickly run out of steam. Pandemics usually come in waves. The 1918 pandemic had three distinct waves—the middle wave was the most lethal—and lasted over a year.

For these reasons, it is vital to set up communication networks from which clear, well-informed information can be disseminated from authoritative sources—and set them up, now.

Current response to H5N1 outbreaks
in the United States

There have as yet been no reported cases of H5N1 outbreaks, in either birds or people in the United States. We are still in surveillance mode.

Responding to outbreaks in birds

The U.S. Department of Agriculture is carefully monitoring H5N1 at its source overseas. According to Dr. Ron DeHaven of the USDA's Animal and Plant Health Inspection Service (APHIS) division, as discussed in a technical briefing on October 25, 2005, "As a primary safeguard, APHIS maintains trade restrictions on the importation of poultry and poultry products from all affected countries. Customs and Border Protection colleagues have been alerted and are vigilantly on the lookout for any poultry or poultry products that might be smuggled into the U.S. from any of the affected countries."

Additionally, USDA quarantines and tests live birds to make sure that pet birds and other fowl from countries not known to be infected don't inadvertently introduce disease into the United States.

These restrictions include: Banning any importation of live birds and hatching eggs from H5N1-affected countries; and mandatory quarantine for all imported birds at a USDA bird-quarantine facility, where they're tested for H5N1 before entering the country.

"Early detection and rapid response is the key to minimize the impact on our poultry production as well as minimize any impact with regard to trade restrictions," Dr. DeHaven added. "We have extensive surveillance programs in place in the United States for avian influenza in poultry. Additionally, our commercial poultry industry is extremely vigilant in applying good biosecurity practices. Biosecurity simply means applying some very practical, common-sense measures to keep from bringing unwanted germs on to the farm or into the poultry houses."

The APHIS has had plenty of experience over the past decades in dealing with viral epidemics in farm birds, with both Low Pathogen Avian Influenza (LPAI) as well as Exotic Newcastle Disease (see chapter

4). As a result, they have detailed reporting and response procedures already in place.

Typically, as soon as there seems to be an outbreak of disease, a cadre of specially trained veterinarians is dispatched from APHIS within four hours to conduct an initial examination and submit samples for testing. In 2002, the USDA Agricultural Research Service (ARS) developed a rapid diagnostic test that can diagnose avian influenza within three hours. For suspected LPAI or HPAI, state-level response teams should be on site within twenty-four hours of a presumptive diagnosis.

Should there be any disease, the affected flocks are destroyed, and quarantines and movement restrictions are imposed until the farms are cleaned and disinfected. Further testing is performed to see if the virus has spread in the vicinity.

A vaccine for either LPAI or HPAI can also be administered to flocks to create a buffer within the region—containing the virus while flocks are being culled—as an added precaution.

In addition, state and federal agencies are monitoring for die-offs among migratory waterfowl. If there is a die-off—and, presumably, the presence of H5N1 in this country—the birds will be tested for influenza viruses. If H5N1 were detected, all local public health, agricultural commissioners, and other local and state agencies would be notified, and the warning for increased surveillance among domestic flocks immediately sent to poultry farmers. The farmers would need to ensure that no wildfowl came into contact with their flocks, and that the flocks would not be transported anywhere.

These plans and precautions have been well thought out, and have worked seamlessly during prior outbreaks of LPAI.

But there are several large hitches. For one, the Food and Agriculture Organization (FAO), part of the United Nations, has claimed that live animal transport (from overcrowded factory farms that are appallingly unhygienic to begin with) may well be one of the prime culprits for the rapid spread of the H5N1 in Asia—but there is little regulation of poultry transportation in America. How are birds moved from factory farms to the processing plants? Who is overseeing their movement?

And for another, if over 100,000 domesticated and wild birds can be smuggled into America each year, as discussed in chapter 4, how can the

APHIS track the movements and health conditions of all these under-the-radar birds, some of whom may be infected with H5N1?

In October 2005, Taiwanese officials found a thousand birds in a container on a freighter, smuggled from China. They tested positive for H5N1. Luckily, none had been removed from the container and put ashore, and all were destroyed.

And in China, the Nanhui District Wild Life Protection and Management Station reported that they'd confiscated more than one hundred bird nets and five hundred wild ducks in the latest raid.

If this can happen in a Taiwanese port and at Chinese beaches, it can just as easily happen here. We have to worry about rogue smugglers as much as we have to worry about a rogue virus.

Responding to outbreaks in people

As I've said, there have been no cases of bird flu in people in this country. So far, there have only been cases in China, Thailand, Cambodia, Vietnam, and Indonesia. It is still assumed that all those infected had contact with birds, although several are being investigated to determine if there had been any person-to-person transmission.

In a discussion about bird flu sponsored by the State Department, Dr. Karen Smith, public health director for Napa County, California, talked about public health strategies to combat bird flu. "In the early stages of a pandemic, when affected areas are localized, some level of surveillance and/or control of persons entering a country from an affected area would likely be one of the measures put in place," she said. "Such measures could range from symptom screening prior to departure and/or upon arrival (as we saw during SARS) [in airports] to canceling flights from affected areas. While some of these measures may have some impact on the spread of the disease, such impact is likely to be temporary."

Hospitals will need to have pandemic plans in place. This necessitates a seamless functioning network of laboratories for testing, and any additional medical training for health-care workers. At present, the test for H5N1 in the laboratory is fairly quick, but specimens still need to be transported to labs. "There is a major push right now to ensure that all the labs in the U.S. Laboratory Response Network—a network of public health labs—have the capacity to do at least the initial typing tests for influenza A and that the higher level labs are doing actual [viral] strain typing," Dr. Smith added. "Few, if any, private labs are set up to do strain typing of influenza viruses."

There are many challenges for pandemic planners. A new report from the Trust for America's Health (TFAH), a public health advocacy group based in Washington, D.C., entitled "A Killer Flu? 'Inevitable' Epidemic Could Kill Millions," found that over 500,000 Americans could die and over 2.3 million could be hospitalized if only a moderately severe strain of a pandemic flu virus strikes. Based on their model estimates, 66.9 million Americans would be at risk of contracting the disease. Of these, over 2 million Americans may need to be hospitalized, and as of the end of 2005, there are only about 965,256 staffed hospital beds in this country.

"A full-blown pandemic could easily mean five hundred hospital admissions every day for six months," said Dr. Irwin Redlener, director of the National Center for Disaster Preparedness. And that's just for New York City, where emergency services and the public health system were tested on 9/11, and vastly improved ever since.

"Responding quickly and effectively to a pandemic requires a comprehensive national plan integrated with state- and local-based emergency planning," TFAH spokesman Michael Earls told me. "Our government hasn't adequately planned for the disruption a flu pandemic could cause to the economy, to daily life, to food and supply distributions, or to homeland security."

The only way to take action to this sobering report is to contact your local and state elected officials. Voice your concerns. Adequate aid did not arrive to many of the victims of Hurricane Katrina when they needed it most. What will happen if a pandemic strikes the entire nation?

ARE HOSPITALS PLANNING FOR A PANDEMIC?

During the SARS scare in 2003, I was on call one weekend when a man walked into the emergency room at the Tisch Hospital at the New York University Medical Center where I am the section chief for infectious diseases. He had symptoms compatible with SARS and had recently returned from Guangdong Province, China, where there had been SARS outbreaks.

Basically, the entire hospital came to a standstill. We had procedures and policies in place, but they had not yet been tested in real-time. We all suited up in protective gear, with N95 masks, suits, and goggles—but were confronted with the need for coordination among the many types of personnel, from health-care providers and students, to housekeepers, building maintenance, and food-service handlers. All of us needed to render care in a compassionate and professional manner, while protecting ourselves, as well as our other patients.

Fortunately, this patient did not have SARS. We used this episode as a learning exercise, and quickly convened a number of committees. We knew we needed to figure out how to prepare ourselves for a similar, potential walking biologic time bomb.

Most large hospitals in metropolitan areas of America have disaster plans and teams in place. Preparedness programs dealing with biological terrorist attacks, enacted after 9/11, will help with pandemic preparedness.

Still, the questions are many: Are these disaster plans up to date, or are they rusty? Have they been used? How often are drills held? What are the isolation procedures? Where will flu-infected patients be placed? (At NYU, we have plans to create segregated wards for flu victims by setting them up in non-clinical parts of the physical plant.)

And what about surge capacity should there be a pandemic where many people become seriously ill at the same time? This could be problematic, as the surge capability in most hospitals is minimal; they run at a very high census, if not over-census. That means they're full—of patients in beds or of patients in the emergency room waiting for a bed. There are rarely open beds in any major hospital.

During a pandemic, we also must be able to deliver vaccines (if there are any) and other treatments to front-line responders and those most at risk. Supplies such as syringes, respirators, masks, and protective equipment would be in short supply. Some of these supplies are being stored as part of the Strategic National Stockpile devised and supervised by the U.S. Department of Health and Human Services.

Unlike viral vaccines, antibiotics for the treatment of secondary infections

> are fairly easy to manufacture. Plus they have a long shelf life and there is a large inventory already in place. Unlike the Tamiflu that must be taken at the first sign of flu symptoms, there is a wide range of choice in antibiotic treatment.

Current response to H5N1 outbreaks outside the United States

Responding to outbreaks in birds

In countries like Vietnam, where there have been many severe outbreaks of bird flu in birds, and forty-two of the ninety-three infected people have died, local and WHO investigators arrive as quickly as possible to allegedly infected areas, and flocks are killed as soon as there are confirmed outbreaks. All other Asian countries where there have been outbreaks have done the same, culling millions of infected and still healthy farm birds. Authorities in Hong Kong, where H5N1 first surfaced, said the government would kill all poultry in the territory if the H5N1 bird flu strain is found in chickens there, and permanently shut down their 2,260 poultry farms.

This is still an extremely complex situation. It's easy enough to cull or vaccinate poultry on large factory farms, where the birds live in enclosed spaces and can be accurately counted. But the vast majority of poultry in Asian countries live on family farms, and the vast majority of these family farms exist at a subsistence level. They have no income to spare. They cannot afford to kill the farm birds that feed their families. Traditionally, birds that are ill are often killed, prepared, and eaten by family members. It's either eat the sick bird, or starve, a concept unimaginable to many Americans who suffer from a daily surfeit of food, not a lack of it.

There is also plenty of overreaction to the H5N1 situation. Birdwatchers are afraid to go out into the field. Some countries have incidents where harmless wild birds are being killed. Although the 43 million domestically reared ducks in Vietnam are much more likely to be infected, a flock of wild ducks near Ho Chi Minh City was recently slaughtered. The Food and Agriculture Organization of the United Nations (FAO) stepped in to stop the killing. "Culling the wild birds is time-consuming and costly, and risks distracting authorities from the real risk, which is the one posed by poultry," said FAO officer Jan Slingenbergh. "Controlling the virus in poultry is the most effective way of limiting the likelihood of the bird flu virus acquiring human-to-human transmissibility."

During a routine check in British Columbia, Canada, in November 2005, LPAI was detected in two commercially reared ducks on two different farms. Although the strain was not lethal and the infected ducks had not become ill, all 65,000 ducks on both farms were culled. Importation of duck from British Columbia was temporary banned by the USDA.

A rather zealous response to LPAI is not the solution for an HPAI like H5N1. It's like trying to eradicate the common cold virus in an attempt to eradicate the flu. It just isn't logical.

Responding to outbreaks in people

The WHO first developed a pandemic plan for human cases in 1999, and updated it in 2005. Their key recommendations for all countries are as follows:

- Strengthen the WHO Global Influenza Surveillance Network to ensure collection, testing, and timely transfer of clinical specimens to one of the four WHO collaborating centers for reference and research on influenza
- Assure prompt and transparent reporting of early human cases
- Develop integrated surveillance systems
- Concentrate on the inter-pandemic phase, to assure early detection of a pandemic strain
- Focus on the ability to detect unusual clusters of respiratory diseases as part of an early warning system
- Use field investigations to determine the characteristics of the virus, follow the dynamics of human-to-human transmission, and identify the specific mutation.

The WHO has also encouraged countries to draft national pandemic preparedness plans, which include holding drills. Drills have already taken place in many countries, including Vietnam, Australia, Taiwan, and

Great Britain. Even the normally secretive North Korea has publicly stated that they've enacted quarantine controls at entry points, are vaccinating some of their poultry, and are monitoring migratory birds.

In November 2005, more than six hundred delegates from over one

---

WILL CHINA TELL US THE TRUTH?

"In 2003, we defeated SARS. That will inspire us to victory over bird flu," claimed Chinese premier, Wen Jiabao.

The initial Chinese denials about SARS, which I discussed in chapter 5, created what could have spiraled into a truly nightmarish situation, and it is heartening that government officials in their tangled bureaucracy are acting with increased transparency about avian influenza, reporting outbreaks more quickly, and with specific numbers. They also set up a nationwide network of emergency offices and plans, as well as mobilizing a national "command headquarters" to coordinate them. On the other hand, officials initially downplayed the disastrous complications after a toxic spill of benzene into the Songhua River in November 2005. Undoing decades of indoctrinated behavior in Chinese bureaucrats is going to be an uphill battle.

China's Ministry of Agriculture issued an "emergency response" for any bird flu outbreaks in animals, demanding that local officials report suspected cases within four hours. "Those responsible for hiding, overlooking or delaying reports will be harshly punished according to the law," Wen Jiabao stated. This is welcome news, as it will encourage local officials to stop hiding incidences of disease, which they were previously encouraged to do. Farmers have also been told that they will be compensated for culled poultry, although they may still incur painful economic losses.

Still, China is so vast, with so many billions of birds, that containing outbreaks may be a losing battle. "Local officials are now paying attention, but there's not much money to build up monitoring," said ornithologist and government advisor Chu Guozhong, "and in some places it hasn't arrived yet."

And the *China Daily* reported that after 2,600 chickens died in twenty-four hours on a farm in Inner Mongolia, more than 90,000 birds within a seven-mile radius were killed. That was the proper response.

Local reporters were forbidden to write about it. That was *not* the proper response.

hundred countries convened at a meeting organized by the World Organization for Animal Health (OIE) in Geneva, Switzerland. They agreed upon a pandemic preparedness plan that would include building and testing national pandemic preparedness plans; conducting a global pandemic response exercise; strengthening the capacity of health systems; training clinicians and health managers; setting up integrated country plans to coordinate technical and financial support; and strengthening communication between nations.

Again, this may sound comprehensive, but the desire to ensure a swift response is often superceded by local customs, abysmal or nonexistent public health departments, and ignorance of what the bird flu truly is. For example, in West Java, Indonesia, two brothers in one family died from what was diagnosed as typhoid fever. When their sixteen-year-old brother also became ill with similar symptoms, only he was tested for H5N1—and turned up positive. Although the family's chickens had died from an illness before the brothers became ill, therefore implying that the transmission of H5N1 was from the birds to people, it's impossible to know if this was indeed a true case of person-to-person transmission. It's too late to test the deceased brothers. An investigative team of WHO and Indonesian health ministry investigators went house-to-house, to all eighty families in the small village, and found no other symptoms in the community.

It's hardly fair to blame the devastated family or the local villagers for not assuming this might have been bird flu.

Even for those well-educated enough about bird flu to summon local authorities to get help, how will poor communities in developing nations procure supplies and medication if there is a local outbreak? How will sick patients be transported to hospitals on unpaved roads? Who will be exposed in the meantime? How will an outbreak be curtailed? Will quarantines be imposed, and if so, how will they be enforced?

"Many countries where the disease is endemic have already taken action," said Dr. Louise Fresco, assistant director-general of the FAO, "but they are overwhelmed by the situation and require urgent assistance."

Who is going to provide that to them?

I can't answer that question. I wish I could.

Part IV

TREATMENTS
and
PROTECTION

Chapter 7.

ALL ABOUT
FLU VACCINES

It is not only possible, but also important, that influenza
pandemic vaccines be made available, and there's a shared
responsibility needed to make that happen. We have a huge
window of opportunity now.

—*WHO influenza program chief Klaus Stohr*

Without question, the best way for a population to stave off a pandemic flu virus is to possess immunity to it.

In other words, our first line of defense against the bird flu is not a pill. It's a vaccine.

The scientific community is working hard to develop a vaccine that could confer some, if not total, immunity to the H5N1 virus. As H5N1's genetic sequence has been decoded, creating this vaccine may be possible. The hitch—and this is a very *large* hitch—is that the current technology of vaccine development and manufacture is arduous, time-consuming, and expensive.

On November 1, 2005, President Bush outlined a $7.1 billion pandemic strategy. His goal is to stockpile enough vaccine to protect 20 million Americans against H5N1, at a cost of $1.2 billion, as quickly as possible. The ultimate goal is, of course, an available vaccine for nearly 300 million Americans. The president also asked for $2.8 billion to speed the development of vaccines based on more effective vaccine-manufacturing technology than what currently exists. (This sum had not yet been approved by Congress as this book went to press.)

"We don't have the capacity to manufacture the vaccine necessary to combat a pandemic," Michael Leavitt, director of the Department of Health and Human Services (HHS, which oversees the CDC), has stated. "We need the ability to isolate a virus and convert it to a vaccine and produce enough vaccine for 300 million people—and we need to do that in six months. That capacity doesn't exist today."

Then again, if it takes many months for a vaccine to be both manufactured and distributed to billions of people around the globe, the virus might mutate so rapidly that any preexisting vaccine may give only partial immunity by the time it *can* be administered.

At which point it may be too late.

An effective vaccine needs to work against the *pandemic* strain—which will undoubtedly differ from the strain that's killing people in Asia now.

ABOUT VACCINES FOR PEOPLE

How does a vaccine work?

Vaccine therapy is an approach to disease prevention that's based on an ingenious strategy. Vaccines stimulate the host's (namely, a person's) immune response into a state of vigilance against specific germs, and in the case of viruses, against specific virus subtypes. They lure the body's immune system into thinking that it's already infected so that it can become activated and fight back right away. (See the section on immune response in chapter 2 for more about this.)

When you receive an inoculation or a nasal spray containing a simile of disease-causing virus—an extraneous antigen that is similar to, if not identical to, some of the components on the actual germ that you're trying to prevent—your body's immune system assumes it's the true intruder. It immediately begins to mount a response. Both cellular as well as antibody responses are created, and they remain active for years, in the ready. Your immune system is, in essence, primed and preactivated for any future assault.

If you are then exposed to the actual germ, your body virtually immediately initiates a cascade of immune defenses, called an amnestic response, including the manufacture of antibodies—instead of waiting the usual week or more it takes for an immune system response to an invader. The small amount of virus that is present during the initial infection won't get a chance to invade its target cells and replicate. Hopefully, this will quell the infection before it can hurt you.

Vaccines may be inactivated (killed) whole virus, or split virus. (See page 124 for an explanation of how a virus is split.) Whole virus vaccines whether inactivated (killed) or attenuated (still able to infect cells but unable to cause disease) are more immunogenic (create a larger immune response) than split virus vaccines. However, whole virus vaccines are generally more toxic, especially to young children.

Vaccine efficacy depends upon a number of factors. First and foremost, only a healthy immune system can recognize a vaccine antigen and develop an effective immune response to it. Therefore, persons with altered immune systems, such as those on chemotherapy, or those with HIV/AIDS, may not respond to vaccines as well as healthier individuals. Similarly, if the immune system is in the midst of dealing with an ongoing illness, such as the common cold or bacterial pneumonia, it may not be able to recognize the small amount of antigen contained within the vaccine, rendering it ineffective. (Your physician would generally choose not to give you a vaccination if you have a fever or are otherwise ill.)

Second, the amount of antigen is critical to the ability of the vaccine to stimulate a protective immune response. The more antigen that is present, the more effective (and possibly the more toxic) the vaccine will be. Sustainable immunity to a vaccine may also require boosters, which are repeat inoculations of the same antigen given to enhance the immune response.

You can also develop immunity to a particular illness after being infected naturally. Millions of people get a mild influenza during the flu season, and will, if they recover, develop immunity to that particular subtype of flu virus. This immunity can last for many years. Cross immunity may also occur in both natural infection and after receiving a vaccination. This means you may develop a partial immunity to a strain of virus that is new to you, but is similar enough to a previously encountered strain that the immune system cannot tell them apart.

What is the ultimate goal of vaccine therapy? The purpose of mass vaccination is to immunologically "prime" the population. That is, to achieve immunity to a specific pathogen (germ) in a significant percentage of the population.

Population immunity will occur when there is sufficient cumulative exposure to both natural virus infection (such as getting the flu), and viral antigens contained within the vaccines. The optimal amount of this protective priming percentage is still unclear where bird flu is concerned, but it is likely that immunity in 50 to 60 percent of the world's population might be required before a bird flu pandemic could be thwarted.

In addition, in vaccines directed at a totally new virus subtype, such as H5N1, a single dose will not result in lasting immunity. A second booster shot would be required within a year or so.

Unfortunately, in the United States, our record of vaccination is not very good. The rate of vaccination in target populations is very disappointing. For seasonal flu, the target populations—the ones with the highest attack rates and mortality rates—are well defined. They include anyone over age sixty-five; children ages six months to two years; and people with underlying chronic ailments (such as asthma, cancer, immune deficiency conditions, and HIV/AIDS). Among these at-risk individuals, probably less than 30 to 40 percent are vaccinated each year. (We do a good deal better for pediatric vaccination since entry into the school systems mandate compliance with the vaccination schedules.) For pandemic flu, obviously the "target" population equals the entire population of the globe, and therefore requires the vaccination of a huge number of people.

How does a seasonal flu vaccine program work?

As viruses are continually mutating, no one vaccine can confer a lifetime of immunity to all of the strains and subtypes of influenza that a person will encounter.

The flu vaccine that you receive each year is a trivalent vaccine, meaning that it contains elements from three different influenza viruses. Because it is a split vaccine (parts of each viral type rather than whole virus), each vaccine contains up to six different H (hemagglutinin) and N (neuraminidase) types. Thus, the seasonal flu shots are designed to confer partial immunity to a variety of different subtypes and strains. This partial immunity may persist for several years, which is why annual vaccine programs are so important. It is only through multiple doses of varying vaccines subtypes that the general population will develop effective cumulative immunity.

The precise viral strains used in each year's vaccine are determined through global surveillance of seasonal influenza cases by the World Health Organization. Estimates as to how the virus will mutate in any given year, called antigenic drift (explained in chapter 2), are made based upon strains that have been recovered from people ill with the flu around the world. The approved 2005–2006 influenza vaccine being distributed in the United States contains two influenza A strains and one influenza B strain: A/New Caledonia/ (H1N1), A/New York/ (H3N2), and B/Jiangsu.

It takes about six to eight months to make a final decision as to the precise components of the next year's influenza vaccine and then roll out enough vaccine production to coincide with the influenza season. (The flu has seasonality, as you know if you've gotten sick around the Christmas holidays. Cold weather brings people indoors, where they share the same air and inhale the same virus-laden droplets.)

After an inoculation, the flu vaccine takes about two weeks to become effective. Physicians often hear patients complain that they got sick with the flu right after getting the shot, which is usually not medically plausible. During those two weeks, it is still possible to become ill with the seasonal flu against which that vaccine is directed, some other strain of the flu, or with another illness that mimics influenza. Flu vaccines provide no protection against influenza-like illnesses caused by other viruses.

In addition, it's important to remember than no vaccine is (or ever will be) 100 percent protective. This is especially true in immunocompromised patients. The immune systems of HIV/AIDS patients may not respond effectively to influenza vaccine because their immune systems are altered. This is why I recommend the influenza vaccine to the HIV-negative significant others of my HIV/AIDS patients.

As stated above, the current 2005–2006 influenza vaccine is a trivalent vaccine, with sub-units to two influenza A strains (H1N1 and H3N2), and one influenza B strain. Each contains a total of 45 micrograms of activate or attenuated virus (15 for each of the trivalent subtypes). This year's shot that protects against H1N1 and H3N2 will also give you partial immunity to previous, slightly similar strains, such as H2N1 or H1N3.

But not to H5N1, the bird flu virus.

Lots of people claim they've never gotten a flu shot, and they've never gotten the flu. Why is the flu shot so important?

It's crucial to understand why the flu vaccine is necessary.

For one thing, flu vaccines work. Over 36,000 people die from the seasonal flu each year, and many of them did not get the shot that could have saved them. It is clear in studies of households where a documented case of influenza has occurred, that those family members who have been vaccinated are highly protected from acquiring infection from their sick housemate.

For another, in any influenza season, there will always be a fairly significant prevalence of people walking around with influenza. Many of these individuals are asymptomatic, and are not even aware that they a spreading their disease to others. By reducing the density of persons carrying and spreading virus, we lessen the chances of epidemic influenza. And preventing influenza also prevents other secondary morbid disease, such as bacterial pneumonia, respiratory failure, cardiac complications, and a wide array of complications due to hospitalization.

When it comes to the current fears of an H5N1 pandemic, there is also a theoretical value to widespread seasonal flu vaccination. If more people get their flu shots and there is a smaller incidence of seasonal influenza, then it is likely the epidemiologists will be able to more readily recognize the onset of an H5N1 pandemic, and hopefully let us respond more effectively.

Let's imagine that there have already been several cases of H5N1 in isolated pockets in your country. Imagine the havoc in an emergency room if ten people came in on a given weekend with a fever of 104 degrees, a deep cough, malaise, and muscle aches. If these patients had already gotten their seasonal flu shots several months earlier, it would be much easier to assume they might have H5N1 and react accordingly.

Controlling an epidemic or controlling epidemic spread requires a high index of suspicion. Hospital emergency rooms are not equipped with electron microscopes to immediately examine viruses in samples taken from patients being treated. Rapid laboratory tests using antibody technology give general results that identify an infection as an influenza virus within an hour or two. Specific subtypes and strains, however, need more complicated tests, performed only by public health laboratories, that can take up to a week or more for accurate results. At which point it may be too late for all those people who've been exposed to the infected patient. Effective triage and quick action by ER nurses and physicians are vital to prevent a pandemic strain of virus from spreading to an unsuspecting group of vulnerable patients who have come to the ER for treatment of non-life-threatening accidents or other medical problems.

The flu vaccine is a marvel of modern medical technology. All vaccines are marvels, actually, and I believe that the bulk of modern medical miracles are vaccine-associated. We haven't had an epidemic of polio or smallpox or mumps or measles for decades in this country, although some appear with terrible regularity in less-developed nations. As a result, many, many people have become cavalierly complacent about vaccines, thinking nothing of how they've transformed society from one in which infants and children routinely died from illnesses we now think of as benign or vanquished to one in which children can grow and thrive without fear of being struck down. It is very frustrating for those of us working on the front lines against viruses to have to combat both disease and ignorance. The raging controversy over the alleged link between the mercury-based vaccine preservative Thimeresol used in many vaccine preparations and autism has caused a reluctance among many to subject their children to time-tested vaccines—despite the lack of scientific evidence linking the preservative to this childhood condition.

The capacity of people to so readily dismiss the benefits of vaccine therapy is an especially dangerous attitude now, when vaccines might be the only safety net we will have if a pandemic strikes. The complacent, I-don't-need-it attitude of many Americans to the recommendation for an annual flu shot also means that profits have been reduced for vaccine manufacture as well as for the development of new vaccine technology—and it has been for decades.

"Influenza vaccine demand drives influenza vaccine supply," said Julie Gerberding, director of the CDC in Congressional testimony on November 9, 2005. "During an influenza pandemic, the existence of influenza vaccine manufacturing facilities functioning at full capacity in the United States will be critically important. The U.S. vaccine supply is particularly fragile; only one of four influenza vaccine manufacturers that sell in the U.S. market makes its vaccine entirely in the United States.

"Another important factor is that public demand for influenza vaccine in the United States varies annually," she added. "Having a steadily increasing demand would provide companies with a reliable, growing market that would be an incentive to increase their vaccine production capacity."

In other words, our government can't buy or try to stockpile flu vaccines if no one can make enough of them. Only the biotech company MedImmune is wholly based in America. The Chiron Corporation is based in Emeryville, California, with a vaccine factory in Liverpool, England. Aventis Pasteur is a French company. GlaxoSmithKline's headquarters is in the UK. The higher the demand, the higher the supply.

Don't let another flu season go by without getting your flu shot!

How are vaccines made?

Most vaccines are still produced with 1950s technology. As the flu vaccine is different every year, fertilized chicken eggs are infected with one of that year's three targeted strains of influenza virus, which then begin to replicate in the eggs' cells. The viruses are harvested, purified, and inactivated before being split by a detergent to release the H (hemagglutinin) and N (neuraminidase) antigens. The three split viruses are combined to make one dose of flu vaccine.

The exact egg count needed? At least a staggering 270 million!

Vaccine manufacture is a slow, difficult process, and requires multiple steps; cell cultivation, inactivation, purification, and packaging. Each step poses a potential bottleneck to production. Also, conditions in the plants must be perfect—a problem that was highlighted in the fall of 2004, when a vaccine manufacturer, Chiron Corporation, discovered bacterial contamination in one of their factories, and the tens of millions of doses that were meant to have been provided to America became unusable.

The problem with this system is obvious: chickens can only lay so many eggs, which have to be provided months in advance. (The egg-based cultivation is also a barrier for those people who are allergic to egg products. They cannot be routinely vaccinated for fear of a serious allergic reaction to the vaccine.) Compound this old-fashioned technique with the reality of H5N1—a virus that kills chickens, and is more lethal to their eggs. In fact, the unchanged H5N1 strains are so toxic to chicken eggs that the cultivation yield is too small. To enhance the ability to cultivate H5N1 in embryonic eggs, the virus must be reverse genetically engineered to make it less toxic to these eggs. In effect, the genetically altered H5N1 virus is devoid of the structure that makes it toxic to the eggs. The virus can then be raised in greater concentrations for the production of human vaccine.

Frankly, a more complex and odious vaccine production process is not what we want to think about since speed is of the essence during a pre-pandemic phase.

What about cell-based technology or genetic engineering instead of vaccines made from chicken eggs?

If there is a pandemic, we'd need nearly 300 million courses of vaccine. Plus we'd need them right away. The hope for this capability lies in what's called a cell-culture technique.

It's not hype to state that cell-cultured vaccines have definite possibilities for the treatment of disease in the future.

During the cell technology process, an influenza virus is overlaid on cells taken from kidneys of African green monkeys (Vero cells) or dogs (MDCK cells). The cells are anchored to tiny, round beads (microcarriers) in a growth media inside large biological reactors. The bioreactors are the growth chambers for the virus. Viruses can replicate much more quickly on these beads in these cells in a laboratory than in eggs. The harvesting procedure is the same as with chicken eggs.

As cell technology doesn't depend on a fresh egg supply and the slow culturing of viruses, it could become essential if a rapid production of vaccine is needed. (Those with egg allergies would also be able to be inoculated, finally.) There's less possibility of the kind of contamination that closed the Chiron Corporation down during the production of the 2004 seasonal flu vaccine. And once the system is perfected, it likely will be easier to ramp up; chickens, after all, don't lay more eggs when there's a pandemic.

But there's the rub—the system is not yet perfected. It's not *close* to being perfected.

In the spring of 2005, HHS awarded a $97-million contract to Sanofi Pasteur to develop cell-based vaccine technology and a plant in the United States. But clinical trials for viable vaccines grown in cell cultures aren't expected for at least another two years.

Even then, there are no guarantees that cell-cultured vaccines would be perfectly viable, or even close to effective. It's assumed they will be. It's too soon to know with any certainty, however.

Genetically engineered vaccines for influenza also have potential, as this technology has proven to be successful for vaccines that provide immunity to other diseases, such as hepatitis B. In this instance, a hepatitis B virus gene coding for its surface coat is inserted into yeast cells. The yeast, saccharomyces, then uses its cellular machinery to produce the antigen, which is later extracted from the cell culture, purified, and used in people. Yeast cells are certainly more abundant than embryonic chicken eggs.

What could also be attempted with a genetically engineered influenza vaccine would be a recreation of a component of the H5 and the N1 proteins. They'd somehow be built and attached to something benign, such as a bacteria; or an inert substance, called an adjuvant, that would help a body's immune system recognize them—and develop antibodies to them, thereby provoking the much-needed immunity.

If this technique worked, hypothetically a monovalent vaccine could be created.

This technology with influenza viruses is, unfortunately, also many years away from being tested and perfected.

Other types of vaccine technology are also being studied. Research studies about DNA vaccines; improved delivery of nasal spray attenuated flu vaccines; and the link between the dominant strain of the flu virus and its effect on the human immune system are ongoing.

What's being done to develop an H5N1 vaccine? How quickly can one be manufactured?

Vaccine production has not been an American priority in recent years. One of the biggest obstacles is litigation from those claiming to have been harmed by vaccine side effects. (See the sidebar on The Swine Flu Vaccine Debacle for more information.) In addition, vaccine development for pharmaceutical companies is just not as lucrative as drug development. Before bringing it to market, first the concept behind a vaccine's creation has to be proven, then it must be tested in strictly supervised clinical trials, then its safety must be assured, then it has to approved by the FDA. Ensuring both efficacy and safety requires large population studies, and this is a very, very difficult process taking many years if not decades. And then there is the problem of tens if not hundreds of millions of development dollars needed to create a new vaccine.

Imagine doing all this, and people still distrust the very life-saving vaccine that has been so carefully tested and regulated.

Since the process for regular vaccine development is so convoluted, and potentially prohibitedly expensive, priority given to a new vaccine to counter bird flu had been slow—until the flu began to spread with alarming rapidity.

According to Tommy Thompson, the former secretary of HHS who was alarmed by reports of bird flu in Asia, requests he made to Congress several years ago to upgrade our vaccine capability from chicken eggs to cell-culture technology were ignored at first. It wasn't until the flu vaccine shortage in the fall of 2004 that $100 million was approved.

In November 2005, President Bush finally admitted that much greater sums—to the tune of $2.8 billion—were immediately needed to help spur progress in new vaccine technology. (At the end of December 2005, Congress had approved only $3.8 billion.)

INCREASING THE FLU VACCINE SUPPLY

There are ways in which the amount of antigen necessary for a good immune response can be "stretched" in a vaccine.

One way is to deliver the vaccine intradermally—under the skin itself, as opposed to the subcutaneous or muscle tissue where a needle is inserted in your upper arm. The skin contains very active antigen-presenting cells, called Langerhans cells. These cells are able to detect "foreign" proteins, and present them to the immune system, which encourages a brisk response.

Less vaccine is needed when given intradermally, than intramuscularly. One study found that one-fifth the dose of standard flu vaccine given intradermally could give the same or a better immune response as the standard shot in the upper-arm muscle. The challenge of intradermal vaccination is that it is technically more difficult to administer, and takes an experienced, steady hand.

Another way that vaccines can be made to be more immunogenic is to chemically attach them to an inert substance, called an adjuvant. An adjuvant is a larger, inert chemical that essentially flags down the immune cells to force them to recognize the antigen, even if present in smaller quantities. As a result, a smaller amount of antigen/adjuvant complex will induce a more brisk immune response. A vaccine given with an adjuvant almost invariably confers a greater degree of response, as well as one with a greater duration. It may also potentially trigger a more complete immune response than the vaccine without the adjuvant

Exactly how much vaccine antigen is required to incite an effective immune response varies. In recent years attention has been refocused on smallpox as a potential agent of bioterrorism. Although there were inadequate stores of vaccine, studies were undertaken by the National Institutes of Health (NIH) that proved that diluting the stored vaccine ten-fold still left an effective immunogen. This is

one way of stretching the store of smallpox vaccine to protect the entire population in this country.

   With H5N1, it is hoped that an adjuvant might lessen the amount of actual
vaccine necessary for immunity. The vaccine manufacturer, Chiron Corporation,
has been testing a vaccine for an older strain of bird flu virus, H9N2, with an adjuvant. They've seen that only one-quarter the usual dose of vaccine plus the adjuvant gave an equivalent antibody level to those tested with the full dose of the
non-adjuvant vaccine.

   Additional studies with adjuvants are underway at the National Institutes of
Health. We should have some idea by the spring of 2006 if adjuvants will work
with the H5N1 vaccine currently being tested.

In the meantime, testing began of an experimental H5N1 vaccine,
made from a killed virus isolated from a patient in Vietnam who'd been
infected by a chicken. The testing has been overseen by the National Institutes of Health (NIH). With funds from the Strategic National Stockpile (SNS), the CDC purchased approximately two million bulk doses of
as-yet unlicensed H5N1 vaccine that still needs to be formulated into
vials. Clinical testing in children and adults, to determine dosage and
schedule for this vaccine, began in April 2005.

   This experimental vaccine hasn't yet been approved for public use.
This doesn't mean it's ineffective, only that the testing process is slow and
cumbersome, as it should be when new drugs and vaccines are being developed for introduction into the population at large. We can presume
that if there is a pandemic, the testing and approval process would be
greatly accelerated by the FDA.

   The experimental vaccine has so far been safe in healthy young patients, and is about to be tested in healthy volunteers over the age of sixty-
five.

   Should H5N1 mutate, as it is expected to do, the experimental vaccine
may still confer limited immunity. Obviously, some immunity is better
than none in a pandemic situation.

   "If there was a true emergency need to vaccinate people, we could
probably use the data we have now and feel pretty comfortable about for-

mulating a vaccine," said John Treanor of the University of Rochester, who's been leading the study.

Still, this experimental vaccine has some major, unexpected drawbacks. "The good news was that the vaccine we developed works. It provides a good immune response that augurs well for protecting people against the H5N1 virus," said CDC director Julie Gerberding in testimony to Congress. "The sobering news was that to achieve the desired immune response, the vaccine needed to be six times as potent as the seasonal vaccine—ninety micrograms of the H (hemagglutinin) component instead of fifteen micrograms—and that two doses are needed for the protective immune response. We need an aggressive strategy to achieve the needed domestic vaccine manufacturing capacity as quickly as possible, and to initiate similarly aggressive action to implement other immediate preparedness strategies beyond these critical vaccine needs."

Even though the vaccine's potency is in question, the CDC plans to stockpile enough doses for 20 million people, at a cost of $162 million. They've given contracts to Sanofi Pasteur and Chiron Corporation to create the vaccine. This sounds promising, but all of these 20 million doses won't be ready for another *four* years. "As we are only able to obtain pre-pandemic vaccine during the few months of the year when influenza vaccine manufacturers are not running at full capacity making the seasonal trivalent vaccine," Gerberding added, "we are severely limited in the quantity of vaccine that we can stockpile."

HHS has also outlined plans to entice the pharmaceutical industry to dramatically increase domestic vaccine production. One of their main efforts is to expand the nation's use of influenza vaccine during interpandemic influenza seasons. Doing so will help assure that the United States is better prepared for a pandemic.

It bears repeating: Get your flu shot!

If there is an immediate investment and expansion of vaccine manufacture, HHS believes that the increased production capacity and related stockpiling capability will be achieved in phases between 2008 and 2013. (That's *seven* years from now.) First of all, they must expand the number of licensed domestic egg-based influenza vaccine manufacturers from the single one that currently exists. It is also hoped the adjuvants may be useful in minimizing the dosage of this vaccine, but several more years of testing are still needed to prove this.

Other countries are, thankfully, working on vaccine development as well. The Chinese company Sinovac Biotech recently announced that it's in the process of developing an alum adjuvanted H5N1 vaccine, called Panflu, for human use. As discussed above, the use of an alum adjuvant may overcome the problems of needing larger amounts of H5N1 antigen, and/or the need for booster shots. They're testing it at extremely low dose levels—as low as 1.25 ug H protein (compared with the 90 ugms required of vaccines produced without adjuvant). The lower the dose needed, obviously, the fewer doses will have to be manufactured, and the more doses there will be for the public. Sinovac's managing director, Yin Weidong, said that testing on one hundred volunteers would take 210 days. After that, it will take a little over four months to manufacture. It's much too early to tell if this vaccine will be effective.

Furthermore, although it's welcome news that vaccine production is being researched and developed around the world, it is highly unlikely that, when confronted with a documented pandemic, any pharmaceutical companies outside the United States would export vaccine to us until *after* they have completely satisfied their own domestic needs.

As it stands now, the challenge is the mass production of a flu vaccine. The heartening news is that it's only been a little over a year since the WHO and other virus watchers have identified that H5N1 was spreading. It took about a month to identify the strain of virus needed to develop a vaccine, and a further three to four months to make this vaccine available to birds. But the bird vaccine, as I'll discuss starting on page 133, is given in a dose far smaller than is needed for people.

The *dis*heartening news is that a number of significant obstacles stand in the way of any rapid roll-out of a bird flu vaccine as was done with the swine flu vaccine in 1976 (see the sidebar on page 134). Large pharmaceutical companies are gun-shy of vaccine development. The expense—running into the hundreds of millions—involves all levels of production: determining which virus, what type of vaccine (whole virus, split virus, adjuvanted), testing for safety and efficacy, overcoming biologic challenges (such as H5N1 lethality to embryonic chicken eggs), ramping up

production facilities, and costs of inventory. And then there is the threat
of litigation; the expense of development is staggering (hundreds of millions of dollars, if not billions); the FDA regulatory process is extremely
rigorous; and there are relatively smaller profit margins compared with
new medications.

In addition, while seasonal vaccine needs to be administered yearly,
investing in vaccine for a *potential* pandemic strain that would only be
required for a brief, albeit vitally important, time frame is especially risky
from a business perspective during an already tough economic climate.

Should a pandemic be announced, the procedure to make a vaccine
would follow several stages. First of all, it is highly doubtful that any vaccine would be available in the early days of a pandemic. Once the infectious strain is genetically identified, the race would be on by
immunologists at the CDC and in other countries on to select the strain
that would offer the most immunity to the pandemic virus. (This is a
compressed form of the procedure the CDC follows each year when
they're deciding what influenza strains to include in the seasonal flu
shot.) Next, the vaccine would be manufactured. This would take a minimum of several months.

And then there are the logistics of providing mass inoculations to a
panicked and undoubtedly by-then-seriously-ill population.

Our country simply must have a production capacity enabling it to
vaccinate the entire population within six months of the onset of a pandemic. This is nowhere close to reality. Even though President Bush's as-yet-
unapproved pandemic plan has allocated $800 million for construction of
vaccine production facilities, this will take many, many years to occur. It's
more of an investment in the future than a response to the immediate
threat of a pandemic.

Not very reassuring, is it?

The single greatest obstacle to preparing for a pandemic is the limited
existing capacity to produce a vaccine. If everyone in the United States
were to be vaccinated against H5N1, 600 million doses (two times the
population of nearly 300 million) would be required. Remember that we
are naïve to this strain of the flu. As an unprimed population, we each
need two shots in order to achieve acceptable complete immunity.

The current production capability for vaccine production in the

United States is 60 million doses each year (for a 45 microgram trivalent vaccine), or 180 million doses (of a 15 microgram monovalent vaccine). It's too soon to know what amount of antigen would be optimal for a new H5N1 vaccine. What we need to have in readiness for the future is a seamlessly functioning vaccine manufacturing capability, so that if there is a pandemic—either with H5N1, or the next virus that mutates into human-to-human transmissibility—we will be ready for it.

We should look back to manufacturing strategies during World War Two to do so. Although culturing viruses is not the same as building tanks and bombers, American ingenuity ought to be focusing on this task. Without a minute to lose.

This could be vital to our survival.

VACCINATING THE AVIAN POPULATION

Birds, and all mammals, can be inoculated to prevent diseases in the same way as humans can. A vaccine for birds, to prevent bird flu viruses, has been in circulation for over a decade. When properly administered with a vaccine "gun" that's more speedy than a needle, a bird flu vaccine in birds is extremely effective. Chicks receive their first shot at the tender age of two weeks, followed by a booster shot four weeks later. (This makes the inoculation process doubly daunting.)

Luckily, a vaccine for birds isn't anywhere as expensive to produce as is a bird flu vaccine for humans—a mere ten cents a dose. (Of course, multiplying that by billions isn't exactly a paltry expense, especially for low-income countries.) It is also possible to produce vast quantities of doses (up to 100 million each day, according to Chinese officials) in a short amount of time, as the necessary dose is a scant one-quarter to one-half a milliliter. Vietnam and Indonesia are in the process of giving vaccines to flocks of their chickens near infected areas. China has already shipped over forty-five tons of bird flu vaccine to Vietnam to help ramp up its inoculation program in farm birds.

To be realistic, however, there are hundreds of millions of domesticated birds in each of the Asian countries, outside of China, hard hit by bird flu. Attempting to catch all of them, one by squawking one, and

THE SWINE FLU VACCINE DEBACLE

Back in 1976, when several cases and one death from swine flu created a panic that this virus was about to mutate into a pandemic, the CDC decided that everyone in this country should be vaccinated—and vaccinated quickly. The National Influenza Immunization Program (NIIP) was created to oversee the manufacture, distribution, and injection of 200 million doses.

It was an extremely complex undertaking. First high-risk groups (hospital patients, nursing home residents, health-care workers) would be vaccinated, in nursing homes and in public health departments. Everyone else would be instructed to line up at schools, factories, medical centers, and shopping centers. Inoculations would be by jet gun instead of the slower, more cumbersome syringe. Mandatory informed consent would allow the tracking of the inoculated as well as potential cases of the flu.

Nothing about this rushed program was easy. Each chicken egg yielded only one dose of vaccine; two had been expected. This delayed production. In the vaccine itself, only the H (hemagglutinin) protein induced an effective antibody response, while the N (neuraminidase) did not. This rendered the vaccine less than optimally viable. Then, it was discovered that the vaccine was least effective in young adults and children.

As more people became inoculated, alarming reports began to surface. A rare, complicated neurological disease, Guillain-Barré syndrome (GBS), was suddenly appearing where it was not expected. Usually, there were only 0.7 cases of GBS per million adults each year. During the NIIP program, there were 8.3 cases per million in those vaccinated.

By the time the NIIP program was summarily shut down in December 1976, twenty-five people had died from GBS and there were an additional five hundred cases, many of these leading to lasting neurological complications in those infected. To top it all off, the seasonal flu was by then making its usual, unwelcome appearance. But because all the vaccine to counteract it had already been melded with the swine flu vaccine—and the swine flu vaccine was effectively banned—no one could then get a flu shot.

In the end, only 24 percent of Americans received a swine flu vaccine. The government, which had assumed all liability for the NIIP, was socked with millions of dollars in lawsuits.

It is in part due to the extremely expensive litigation after this debacle that few drug companies (and their shareholders) currently believe it's worthwhile to develop and sell vaccines—especially as American citizens are far more litigious now than they were in the 1970s.

For this reason, President Bush stated in his pandemic plan that all vaccine manufacturers be absolved of any liability during the development and administration of bird flu vaccines for an upcoming pandemic. This may sound only fair, should we be desperate and clamoring for vaccine while people are dying from the flu. But what if the experimental vaccine currently being tested, or another vaccine as yet to be developed, turns out to have lethal side effects? Who should be held responsible? Does a global disaster caused by one disease preclude public safety on other issues surrounding this disease? These are tough ethical questions to answer.

guarantee that the entire population has been vaccinated, is a daunting if not impossible task. Many of the chickens and ducks raised in Asia belong to rural farming families, and they run freely in yards and into houses. They aren't caged in large factory farms, where there can be an accurate head count, as they are in America. Inspecting and monitoring the vaccination process will be a logistical nightmare, to put it mildly. And workers are often poorly trained, if not inadvertently negligent. Not all of them wear protective gloves when handling poultry; syringes are improperly discarded; feces can be spread into homes and other farms; and the attitude toward the seriousness of the situation may not be optimal.

China is home to the largest population of farm birds in the world, almost 21 percent of the world's total. Many provinces in China have been riddled with outbreaks of avian flu over the last few years; there were over fifty outbreaks in sixteen provinces last year, and infections have been reported in almost every province since mid-October 2005. The first of three bird flu deaths in people occurred in November 2005. Hundreds of thousands of birds have already been culled.

On November 15, 2005, Chinese officials stunned the world when they announced an ambitious program. They plan to vaccinate their entire stock of poultry against bird flu. There are 14 *billion* chickens, ducks, geese, and turkeys in China. Yes, 14 *billion*. The government has vowed to succeed, starting at first with 5.2 billion birds, and then ramping up to each and every bird. They plan to pay for this massive undertaking through the central government, supplemented with funds from local provinces.

This is a welcome change from the secrecy of the Chinese government during the SARS epidemic, when they initially denied that anyone was sick with the virus. However, fears are mounting that the program will be both unfeasible as well as potentially riddled with fraud. Fake vaccines for poultry have already been discovered. Worse, some of the fake vaccines may have inadvertently contained actual infectious virus, which would have greatly intensified the ease of its spread. In addition, diluted or otherwise irregular vaccinations could facilitate the breeding of a drug-resistant form of the virus, or mask its symptoms.

The China News Service reported that the State Administration of Industry and Commerce there issued an urgent notice to all its branches, insisting that they swiftly arrest and prosecute anyone selling the bogus vaccines. This has already happened—at the end of November 2005, Chinese police discovered that two companies in Inner Mongolia had manufactured vaccine without a proper license and sold 200,000 vials of twelve different kinds of bird flu vaccine throughout China. Some of the fake vaccines were sent to the Jinzhou area of Liaoning Province, where farms are tightly clustered, making it easier for the virus to spread. Farmers were crushed when over 2.5 million poultry had to be culled as a precaution.

The Food and Agriculture Organization (FAO), a United Nations agency, has stated that they support the Chinese vaccination program, but warned that Chinese-manufactured bird flu vaccines must be subjected to rigorous quality control. (Chinese drugs are not always manufactured under optimal conditions, and can be contaminated with other toxic substances as well as calibrated in dosages below required levels.) This is a problem that is, sadly, endemic in certain areas of the world, where regulation is lax and animal vaccines are not regarded as a top public health priority. Some of the bird vaccines are so diluted as to be next to useless.

It is "absolutely necessary to control the vaccines in a proper manner,"

said the FAO's head of veterinary services, Joseph Domenech. "The quality controls must be done in independent laboratories, not in laboratories
where the vaccines are produced," he said.

Even if the quality of the vaccines in Asia can eventually be assured,
one other factor is guaranteed. It will always be impossible to vaccinate
the wild birds that migrate every year, land in local ponds and lakes, scavenge local food and water supplies, and shed virus in their secretions and
their excrement. As long as flocks of wild birds continue to become infected, and show no signs of these infections (giving no hint that they are
carriers of disease), entire populations of newly hatched, nonvaccinated
farm birds are likely be infected as well.

Still, ambitious hopes and plans to vaccinate billions of birds are
nothing to scoff at. If it's possible to affect the primary concentration of
the virus in the poultry population in any way possible, then we might
just be able to stem the tide of H5N1. Attempting to decrease the density
of the virus within that population of birds is a wise move.

When it comes to animals that fly, however, it's all about chance.
There are so many billions of birds and chickens in the world, and the
more they become infected with a specific virus, the greater the likelihood is that the wrong thing is going to happen. If there is a one-in-
a-million chance of mutation, and you've still got several billion Chinese
chickens that haven't gotten their vaccines yet, anything can happen.

Chapter 8.

ALL ABOUT
FLU DRUGS

Anti-virals are an important part of a comprehensive plan, but
to focus on any one anti-viral is misplaced. There is no certainty
that they will be effective, and, as viruses mutate, there's no
capacity to change the anti-virals to match the virus.
—*David Leavitt, secretary of the U.S. Department of
Health and Human Services*

When the anthrax scare spread in the scary days after the attacks on 9/11, there was understandable panic. Americans had never faced such a real fear of an attack by a biological agent before. At the time, the buzzword was Cipro, a potent antibiotic for the treatment of anthrax. Across the country, many people demanded prescriptions from their beleaguered physicians, hoarded it, and took it although they had no symptoms—or even the remotest possibility of any exposure to potential pathogens. When that happened, they often found that instead of combating anthrax, they were combating some unpleasant side effects from potent medication they didn't need in the first place.

The current buzzword for H5N1 bird flu treatment is Tamiflu, an anti-viral drug. It has been proven to work in some of the patients who were recently infected in Asia—so far, at least. As a result, there's a global shortage as the Swiss manufacturer, Roche Holdings A.G., scrambles to produce hundreds of millions of new doses; governments struggle to

HOW DO ANTI-INFLUENZA DRUGS WORK?

There are two currently available classes of drugs active against influenza:

1. The neuraminidase (N) inhibitors—Tamiflu™ (oseltamivir) and Relenza™ (zanamivir)
2. The M-2 protein inhibitors—Symmetrel™ (amantadine), and Flumadine™ (rimantadine).

The N-inhibitors Tamiflu and Relenza interfere with the viral neuraminidase enzymes that, you will recall, are found on the surface of the virion. The N enzymes are critical in allowing the virus to release from their binding sites on the cell membrane as they enter, and then as the newly formed particles leave the host cell. In the presence of these anti-viral drugs, the replicating viruses cannot exit from the infected cell. Instead, they actually clump together, preventing further cellular invasion. As a result, Tamiflu puts a damper on the rate at which new viral progeny are available to infected healthy respiratory cells. (The N enzymes may also help the influenza virus make its way through the thick respiratory mucus, which is also rich in sialic acids.) By slowing the rate of cellular infection, the body's immune system will have more time to kick in and mount a response to the viral attack.

The N-inhibitor drugs have been licensed for use against Type A influenza in the United States and Europe since 1999. Tamiflu is available as a pill or in liquid form, and Relenza is available as a nasal spray with a special inhaler, which makes it slightly less effective than Tamiflu, as it isn't absorbed directly into the bloodstream.

Studies of effectiveness of Tamiflu against the H5N1 virus in animals have been encouraging, although it seems that higher doses and longer treatment courses might be necessary, compared with those used in seasonal flu treatment. Tamiflu has also been used to treat some of the humans infected with H5N1 avian flu.

The M-2 inhibitors are the older class of influenza therapies. They interfere with the functioning of the M-2 protein, normally located inside the viral coat. This viral protein is critical in the transport of the viral genome from the virus, into the host cell nucleus, where the genetic replication occurs. While active against many influenza A subtypes and strains that cause seasonal flu, they have little or no activity against the H5N1 subtype.

purchase the needed doses for their citizens; and those with access to a generous physician beg, plead, and wheedle for a prescription, so that those who may be already sick with the seasonal flu this year will find it in potentially life-threatening short supply.

Many of my patients, as well as my colleagues' patients, are falling prey to the panic-hoarding frenzy we faced with Cipro and anthrax. They're frantic. They're demanding Tamiflu and they don't even know what it is. All they know is that it's hard if not impossible to procure, and they're afraid they won't be able to get it if indeed there is a pandemic. In the first eight months of 2005, 1.7 million prescriptions of Tamiflu were filled in the United States, a three-fold increase over last year's rate.

WHEN SHOULD ANTI-VIRAL THERAPY BE USED?

The goals of anti-viral therapy for influenza are two-fold. In those who have fallen ill with influenza, treatment can help reduce the severity of symptoms as well as their duration by up to two days, help prevent complications, as well as lessen contagiousness. *But only when the treatment is begun in the first day or two of illness.*

The anti-viral drugs can also be used for prevention of infection, and different strategies have been employed in this manner. The clearest indications seem to be in households where someone already has a documented case of influenza A. At that point, Tamiflu could be prescribed for the healthy family members for five days, until the infectious period of the sick patient has ended.

Anti-viral drug prevention has also been used for those who are employed in nursing homes, or hospitals, to quell outbreaks. They're also helpful for patients at risk for serious seasonal influenza, but who are allergic to egg products and cannot take the vaccine. These persons may take the preventative drugs for the entire flu season!

The important thing to remember with anti-virals is that they are *not* cures for the flu. They can, at their best, limit the damage wrought by the influenza virus until the body's own immune response can do the final clean-up.

Viruses can also mutate, which may lessen their vulnerability to the anti-viral agents. Two of those who died from bird flu in Vietnam had developed resistance to Tamiflu. If H5N1 mutates and gains the ability to be transmitted easily between humans, we are holding our collective breaths, hoping that Tamiflu will remain a plausible therapy. It would be an unkind act of nature if the same H5N1 mutations that turn the virus into a human pathogen also rendered it resistant to Tamiflu.

Is Tamiflu safe?

Anti-virals usually don't have serious side effects. Tamiflu may cause minor adverse reactions such as gastrointestinal distress (nausea and vomiting, diarrhea, dizziness, and insomnia may occur in less that 5 percent of patients). These are usually lessened if Tamiflu is taken with food.

No child under the age of one should be given anti-viral medications.

Tamiflu has been tested and approved for use over a five-day course, and is considered a relatively benign drug with few serious side effects, especially in comparison to antibiotics. There have been infrequent reports of skin conditions in children.

There was, however, a recent scare in Japan, the world's largest consumer of Tamiflu (they usually buy 60 to 70 percent of available doses). Twelve children died after taking Tamiflu. Of these twelve, there were single cases of suicide, pneumonia, asphyxiation, and acute pancreatitis; four cases of sudden death; and four cases of cardiac arrest. In addition, the FDA is investigating thirty-two "psychiatric events," such as hallucinations and abnormal behavior, in children who'd taken Tamiflu. (All but one of these children lived in Japan.) Two of these thirty-two children committed suicide.

Roche claimed that "there is no increase in deaths and neuropsychiatric events in patients on Tamiflu versus influenza patients in general." After an investigation, made more difficult as it was extremely hard to determine whether the children had preexisting conditions exacerbated by the flu, the FDA concurred. They stated that "insufficient evidence to establish that deaths and neuropsychiatric events represent a safety signal associated with Tamiflu."

There have not been any similar reports of psychiatric problems in children taking Tamiflu in the United States. However, we must always be wary about toxicity that occurs at low prevalence, which may remain below the detection of the FDA's "radar screen" until more widespread use of the drug is practiced.

Although millions of doses of Tamiflu have been safely taken in the last few years, often by large groups of people, such as nursing home residents, over a period of several weeks, it has not been tested for long-term use.

And that could become an additional health hazard.

If there is a pandemic, Tamiflu is the type of drug that must be taken continuously during the length of the outbreak in order to remain effective. As pandemics can last for months, this means you, and everyone in your family, would need to keep taking Tamiflu every day for months until reassurance is provided that the danger is over.

Not only is this impractical, it is most likely impossible. There's already a global shortage of Tamiflu, and the amount needed to protect every family in this country over the course of a pandemic is astronomical.

In addition, Tamiflu has not been tested for use over a course of several months. We have no idea of its potential long-term effects; or if indeed it would remain effective for that long. Of course, if there is a pandemic, I should think that most people would be far more worried about dying from the flu than about the hypothetical possibility of damage from long-term use of an anti-viral drug.

There's another point to consider. Let's say the worst-case scenario begins to unfold, and a bird flu pandemic is declared. Local officials doubt they can work, but quarantines are imposed in your town anyway, and all public meetings are banned. You're confined to the house, thankful to have Tamiflu on hand, all things considered, when you begin to feel the dreaded symptoms of the flu coming on. But is it bird flu, or regular flu? Or could it possibly be something else? If you take Tamiflu, and it turns out you didn't have bird flu, you've wasted the treatment. If you wait too long, the drug would be ineffective anyway. If that was your only supply of the drug, and there's no possibility of procuring any more of it, what will you do if the bird flu does strike?

I certainly hope we won't get to the point where there will be a pandemic, or an attempt to quarantine millions of people in large metropolitan areas, or people playing Russian roulette with their desperately hoarded Tamiflu supply. If Roche can successfully gear up its production of Tamiflu, an optimal scenario might be to set up large regional supplies for use in outbreak containment, as well as distributing several days' supplies to each household. Patients with confirmed cases could then rapidly begin therapy without delay, while regional supplies are mobilized to health-care centers or other appropriate facilities.

How could Tamiflu be used in the event of an H5N1 pandemic?

It is safe to say that if a pandemic steamrolls upon us in the manner that the 1918 pandemic occurred, Tamiflu would be of little or no usefulness. However, 1918 was a worst-case scenario. For a variety of reasons, we are more likely to recognize human clusters of infection, and be able to establish a pre-pandemic phase (WHO alerts at Stages 4 and 5). Anti-virals might have critical roles in preventing a full-scale pandemic.

The first way is *prophylactic*. Consider a patient (let's call him Patient X) who arrives in a New York City emergency room with a bad case of what appears to be the flu. Because of prior alert, the triage staff carefully questions Patient X and learns that a week earlier he was in a village in China where human-to-human cases had been identified. Patient X is immediately placed in respiratory isolation. However, the damage may have already been done while he was waiting in the holding area. The infection control staff moves into action, and attempts to identify the staff, other patients, and visitors that may have come in close contact with Patient X. Each potentially exposed person would then be prescribed Tamiflu, advised to remain at home for a period of seven to ten days, and to seek immediate medical attention should flu symptoms develop. Such quick action might avert a rather rapid outbreak.

A similar scenario could unfold on an airplane. If someone became seriously ill with the bird flu two days after getting off a plane, it is possible to check the manifests and track down the other passengers sitting nearby. Modern ventilation systems in jet airliners exchange and filter air very efficiently. It has been determined that a passenger with an illness that spreads via the respiratory route would not be expected to infect other passengers sitting beyond five rows away. Those proximate passengers would be prescribed Tamiflu as prophylaxis.

The caveats in considering the role of prophylactic Tamiflu in these theoretical scenarios are that the optimal duration and dosages might differ for H5N1 than for other influenza A subtypes and strains. (There haven't been enough cases of H5N1 infection in people to test these dose levels yet.) In addition, there may be an increased risk of side effects if higher dosages are required. And, of course, there must be an adequate supply of the drug for rapid deployment.

The second way anti-virals would be used in pre-pandemic and pandemic situations would of course be for *treatment*. In the treatment of seasonal influenza, Tamiflu is effective if begun within the first two days of symptoms. As you read in chapter 1, healthy soldiers in 1918 died within one to two days of the onset of symptoms. How does a physician decide whom to treat with the drug, especially when it is likely to be in limited supply? Health-care providers will need to triage their patients, to determine who is likely to benefit, and who is likely to die regardless of treatment, just as battlefield medics are called upon to perform this very difficult task. If you think about it, a patient presenting on day one or two of illness, who is not exhibiting any signs of respiratory failure, is most likely to benefit from Tamiflu therapy. A patient ill for the same number of days, who requires a respirator, is flushed with heliotrope cyanosis, and is near death, is highly unlikely to benefit, and the drug might rightfully be withheld if supplies were limited. Alternatively, a person seen on day four or five of their illness, who is beginning to improve on his or her own, would similarly not benefit from therapy. These are some of the difficult decisions that need to be made in crisis situations.

Can we be certain the Tamiflu will remain effective should there be a pandemic?

Unfortunately, we can't. It might not be effective in the slightest. Putting the ongoing debate about Roche's proprietary manufacture of Tamiflu aside, the entire discussion might be rendered moot should H5N1 develop a resistance to it in upcoming years or months, as it had in several recent cases in Vietnam. And indiscriminant use of Tamiflu in the global community will exert just the kind of evolutionary pressure the virus needs to acquire mechanisms to resist the anti-viral effects of the drug. Stockpiling Tamiflu commits a lot of sorely needed resources to what might become a stockpile of ineffective medication.

Although N-inhibitors in theory should continue to prevent the entry of viruses into host cells, any highly adaptable virus might find a way to circumvent the N-inhibitor's unique properties. As mutations are impossible to predict, resistance to an anti-viral drug is a definite possibility.

This has already happened during a study sponsored by the National Institute of Allergies and Infectious Diseases of fifty Japanese children who took Tamiflu. It was discovered that there were mutations on the N gene in nine of the children (18 percent)—and all these mutations were Tamiflu-resistant.

It has also already happened with the older class of anti-virals, the M-2 inhibitors, amantadine and rimantadine. They have proven to be completely ineffective on some H5N1 patients in Vietnam.

On the other hand, it is always theoretically possible that the older drugs may become useful against H5N1 if it shifts in such a way that they can effectively treat it.

Why is there a Tamiflu shortage?

The World Health Organization (WHO) recently suggested that every country should stockpile enough Tamiflu to treat at least a quarter of their population. This amounts to a minimum of twenty *billion* doses. As things stand right now, this is an impossible task.

Roche holds the license for Tamiflu, bought from its creators, Gilead Science, over a decade ago. Their patent expires in 2016; until then, anyone who wishes to manufacture Tamiflu must do so with Roche's permission, and pay for the privilege. Roche has invested tens of millions of dollars in its development and manufacture in twelve different factories, which is a complicated, ten-step process that takes over a year, in part because of the hazardous use of sodium azide (the chemical that prompts airbags to explode). Roche claims that this difficult manufacture has been one of the reasons they've been loathe to license Tamiflu's production by other drug manufacturers.

Doubtless they have also been loathe as Tamiflu has turned out to be extremely profitable. Currently, a five-dose prescription carries a pharmacy price tag of between eighty and ninety dollars in the United States. It is discounted to countries that can't afford the wholesale price, and they've donated three million adult courses to the WHO, which will be available by mid-2006.

The active ingredient in Tamiflu, shikimic acid, is extracted from star anise, a spice grown predominantly in China. Due to overwhelming demand, the star anise supply has become limited, which is a worry as Roche depends on it for two-thirds of its Tamiflu manufacture. The other third is derived from fermented *E. coli* bacteria.

Roche has claimed that they hope to reverse that ratio, but they are as yet unable to say when that might happen. They *have* responded to the H5N1 crisis by quadrupling their manufacturing capacity, but as things currently stand, it may take another decade for enough Tamiflu to be available to treat only 20 percent of the world's population. Right now, they can make 55 million treatment courses a year. They hope to ramp up to 150 million courses in 2006 and 300 million in 2007 (less than 5 percent of the world's population).

Roche is in talks with potential partners to license Tamiflu's manufacture, and in December 2005 they agreed to allow fifteen generic drug manufacturers to produce it. This will increase annual production from 27 million to more than 300 million doses by December 2006. This is excellent news. In addition, should there be a pandemic crisis, the World Trade Organization has rules stating that countries can issue compulsory licenses to disregard patents rights (after negotiations and compensation for the patent holder), and these rules can be enforced. In other words, other companies would be able to make Tamiflu during a crisis, but by the time they set up their system for doing so, it might already be too late.

This is a touchy situation. The Indian government, for example, has already stated they're considering invoking a "special law" in which they could circumvent the licensing process to create a generic version of

Tamiflu. And as there's no patent protection for Tamiflu in Indonesia, where there are increasingly prevalent outbreaks. Roche granted permission for that country to begin manufacture without a license. They're about to do the same for Vietnam.

I can't say that I blame Indian officials for putting pressure on Roche. There should be incentives for them to grossly increase their production, as they have fine-tuned the complicated manufacturing process, and they can guarantee that each dose is standardized—something that a generic, quickly made drug might not be able to match. Nor might other factories have a surge capacity, and be able to make any doses in the time needed to stave a pandemic.

If Roche can make a pill for every person who needs it, they should be allowed to. If they need government support and incentives, they should be given. During World War II, the productive capacity of our factories was increased to capacities that would have been unimaginable only a few years before the war started. The airplanes, tanks, and munitions *had* to be made. Penicillin also needed to be mass-produced for the treatment of wounded soldiers. We got the job done. A lot of people made a lot of money doing so, too. This is how the business world works.

However, my prime concern is the health and welfare of the population. When AIDS became a crisis situation, I often attended international conferences, and argued with my colleagues that global health should be considered as a sort of eminent domain, that there shouldn't be any patents on drug manufacture during a crisis, and that a developing catastrophe precluded the normal operation of free enterprise. Not surprisingly, many did not agree with me.

Of course, any company's financial interest, regardless of how large a company it is, will pall in the face of the devastating financial impact of an unfettered pandemic.

The CDC (Centers for Disease Control and Prevention) is responsible for procuring Tamiflu for its Strategic National Stockpile (SNS) in the United States. By the end of November 2005, the SNS had approximately 5.5 million adult treatment doses and 110,000 child treatment doses, along with 84,000 treatment regimens of Relenza, on hand. This is hardly enough to treat the barest minimum of those who'd need it first (health-care workers who'd be confronted with a large amount of very sick people in a short time frame, and essential service providers). The population of our country is, after all, over 296 million.

The federal government has announced plans to spend $1.4 billion to buy 20 million more courses of Tamiflu by end of 2006, with a goal of 81 million courses by mid-2007. Of these, 75 million courses would be for the general population, and 6 million would be specially stockpiled to try to contain an initial outbreak. However, that's still not enough for everyone in this country. The recommendation of the Infectious Diseases Society of America is that an ideal stockpile should cover at least 40 percent of the population; 75 million doses only cover about 25 percent.

Part of the $1.4 billion would appropriated for accelerated work on creating new anti-viral drug treatments. "To facilitate the development of new anti-virals, HHS will collaborate with industrial organizations to develop, obtain approval, and establish commercial production of new anti-virals that would help protect the citizens of our Nation," Michael Leavitt, head of the Health and Human Services (HHS) department, said in testimony to a committee in the House of Representatives.

Is that why Tamiflu should not be hoarded?

No drug should ever be hoarded. For one thing, drugs have a use-by date for a reason—they expire, and expired drugs might lead to unforeseen reactions. For another, those who hoard tend to be those who self-diagnose and self-medicate, which can be extremely dangerous.

Plus, any overuse of *any* drug contributes to the growth of resistant strains of viruses and bacteria.

Furthermore, and even more important, Tamiflu is *not* and will *never* be the primary weapon in the fight against a bird flu virus. That primary weapon is a vaccine, as I discussed in the last chapter.

"I think it's a complete misdirection of energy to be so focused on the issue of stockpiling," CDC director Julie Gerberding said, and I agree. "There is no evidence that it will make a difference if we are hit with a pandemic."

DRUG SYNERGISM

When certain drugs are taken in combination, they may be able to enhance each other's action or effectiveness—more so than if taken separately. This is referred to as drug synergism.

During World War II, when penicillin was desperately needed, scientists discovered that another drug used to treat gout, probenecid, effectively blocked the kidney's rapid filtering of the antibiotic. Less was excreted in the urine; therefore more stayed in the body over a longer time period to kill bacteria.

In some studies, when Tamiflu is taken with probenecid, the number of hours its active ingredient works nearly doubles. If this technique works, only half the regular dose of Tamiflu might be needed. That would drastically increase the amount of available doses.

It's not yet known if a Tamiflu/probenecid combination might work during a pandemic. Nor is this combination sanctioned by Roche, or the FDA, as there's not yet enough clinical data to support the use of the combination. It is certain that there will be further studies of existing drugs that might improve the effects of the anti-viral agents already at our disposal.

For those who insist on hoarding their Tamiflu because they need to feel assured that they have something on hand to treat bird flu, this is not likely to be extremely reassuring.

Tamiflu will be most useful to help contain a pandemic while it is still in its infancy, at the localized outbreak stage. That would most likely be in Southeast Asia, where people are currently becoming infected with H5N1. The WHO would have to respond to any potentially epidemic-sized outbreaks with methodical, comprehensive swiftness to keep the virus from spreading. They would have an extremely limited time frame in which to do so—only a few weeks. Any more than that, and containment will fail.

OTHER POTENTIAL MEDICAL APPROACHES
TO THE TREATMENT OF AVIAN INFLUENZA

I have devoted a large portion of this chapter to Tamiflu simply because it is our best available drug at the moment. However, as scientists begin thinking about the H5N1 problem, clinical ingenuity will undoubtedly spur new approaches and tools for treatment.

If you recall how influenza makes you ill (in chapter 2), you will appreciate that the immune system is a "double-edged sword." What I mean by this is that although the immune system ultimately eradicates the virus (if the patient lives long enough), it is also the immune response that causes the tissue damage, which can result in death. Our immune system is a complex array of components; some components are assigned to create highly specific antibodies against the infecting viral strain, and other components produce more generalized inflammatory responses. Cytokines are chemicals released by certain immune cells, called lymphocytes, designed to modulate the immune response. However, in the case of a severe influenza, a "cytokine storm" develops. Patients drown in inflammatory secretions, and organ systems fail due to inflammatory disruption of normal biologic function.

The pandemic of 1918 began in young, healthy people. Many of them were soldiers housed in close quarters, in conditions of questionable hygiene. It was initially put forth the pandemic flu attacked them because they were made vulnerable hosts by their circumstances. They *were* especially vulnerable, of course, but we also know that the pandemic began simultaneously in all corners of the globe. Even in locales not at war, young healthy people fell prey to the disease. It may well have been the vigor of their immune responses to the 1918 influenza that placed them at highest risk.

I attended a lecture given by Dr. David Fedson on November 17, 2005. Dr. Fedson has been a recognized expert in the area of vaccines and was the former head of medical affairs for Aventis Pasteur, a leading vaccine maker. At that conference, he discussed some interesting observations regarding the use of statin drugs (used to control high cholesterol) and influenza. There have been three recent population studies suggesting protective effect from statins, being taken for high cholesterol, against the severe complications of influenza. Now, most people who take statins are in the older age groups, and have other serious health problems. This is the group of people that should have had the highest mortality from seasonal influenza. However, the statin patients had lower incidences of markers associated with influenza mortality. No factor, other than the use of statins, could account for these results. Why would this be?

One possible explanation is that the statins inhibit the pro-inflammatory cytokines. In the coronary arteries, statins may help clear blocked vessels by reducing circulating cholesterol, but also by quieting down the local inflammation in the cholesterol-laden plaques. Neurologists are beginning to look at the statins as a possible treatment for Alzheimer's dementia, a disease thought to be driven by pro-inflammatory cytokines. So, on a hopeful note, if statins prove to modify the influenza-induced "cytokine storm," they may be helpful as adjunctive therapy in the event of a pandemic. Plus, they are abundant, easy to produce, and relatively inexpensive!

In recent years a whole host of cytokine inhibitor drugs have been approved for the treatment of septicemia, autoimmune and rheumatic diseases, certain infections, and organ transplant rejection. It is possible that some of these drugs might assume a role in the treatment of severe influenza infection as well.

Another theoretically promising treatment is passive immunization. This refers to the prevention or treatment of disease by the transfer of antibodies made by one (immune) person into a nonimmune person.

It has been clear since experiments performed in the early 1930s that antibodies protect mice from influenza infection. The antibodies must be specific for the viral subtype/strain, and must be present prior to the infection. Our current use of vaccines capitalizes on this early work by promoting protective antibodies in previously nonimmune persons. But we don't have a vaccine for H5N1 yet.

In 1918, it is likely that more than 50 percent of the entire population of the world had to have been infected and become immune to the pandemic flu virus *before* the pandemic died out. (It took three waves of devastation over fifteen months for this to occur.) Most of those infected were asymptomatic, or mildly ill. Theoretically, and had the technology of the time allowed it, serum taken from people surviving the first wave of the epidemic would have been expected to have high levels of specific antibody against the pandemic virus. Could it have been helpful in preventing the subsequent waves of influenza? Moreover, could the sera of recovered persons been used to treat patients dying of influenza?

This may not be as moot a set of questions as first it appears. In Asia, there have been 142 human cases of H5N1. What we do not yet know is the actual *prevalence* of infection. In other words, there may be hundreds or even thousands of people who have been exposed to H5N1 but never fell ill, yet have developed protective antibodies on their own. Is there a potential source of immune globulin that could be harvested and stored in the event of a pandemic? This is an intriguing concept, and one that deserves further study.

ALTERNATIVE DRUG TREATMENTS

I am not a proponent of alternative drug "cures" for the flu, such as homeopathy and herbal preparations, but many others (including some of my patients) swear by them. If you are interested in alternative and naturopathic medicine, I suggest you have a consultation with a reputable, licensed practitioner who will take a detailed medical history, and carefully explain what is being diagnosed and what is being dispensed to treat it. You must tell this practitioner about any current medications, as there might be contraindications and unwanted interaction.

One of the least sensible things you can do to your body is self-diagnose any illness, and self-treat it with herbs and other potions. Although many Chinese herbs do have medicinal properties, they can also be dangerous unless prescribed by a qualified herbalist and in doses that are standardized and quality-assured. (Some herbal supplements manufactured abroad have dangerous levels of lead, among other compounds.) Not only will they not do anything to treat the flu, but they might make you seriously ill. I've seen plenty of allergic reactions to allegedly "safe" homeopathic medications, which do have active ingredients.

Currently, several double-blind, controlled studies are underway to test the efficacy of several herbal compounds, including elderberry syrup (Sambucol), the anti-inflammatory and antioxidant n-acetylcysteine (Mucomyst, available only by prescription), and American ginseng (CTV-E002). Results are promising, but as I said, these are not cures. At best, they may help relieve symptoms and lessen the duration of the flu. Obviously, none of these compounds has yet been tested for use against the H5N1 virus.

Chapter 9.

PROTECTION
from and
PREPARATION
for the FLU

If a pandemic hits our shores, it will affect almost every sector of our society, not just health care but transportation systems, workplaces, schools, public safety, and more," Michael Leavitt, head of the Department of Health and Human Services has stated, with much needed candor. "We are inadequately prepared."

Lots of people read his words and became very frightened about the possibility of a pandemic. Some physicians and health-care workers are instructing their patients on survival skills, tantamount to turning their rec rooms into intensive care units. One physician in Georgia has even given instructions on conserving Tamiflu by collecting the excreted drug in urine, and "refeeding" it by nasogastric tube to critically ill family members! He means well, but I believe that such doomsday scenarios serve only to panic, not prepare people.

The best way to prepare for an influenza pandemic is to be informed about the biology of the disease. When you are, you'll be able practice preventative measures—*the* most important aspect of dealing with the flu—as well as recognize warning signs early, and seek appropriate medical care when indicated.

And you certainly know by now that **receiving a seasonal flu shot is a must.**

The worst way to prepare for a pandemic is to believe the scaremongers, happy to prey on your fears and your pocketbooks. Just as bad is to bury your head in the sand, and believe that a pandemic of the scale seen in 1918 could never again occur. Believe me, it *could.* As long as there are living creatures, there will be viruses to make them ill. Pandemics happen. They always have and they always will.

I see this pre-pandemic phase as an opportunity to educate yourself about the flu (which you're already doing if you're reading this book), to stock up on household supplies that you should have on hand anyway in readiness for natural disasters or a biological terror attack, and to get vital paperwork such as wills and insurance in order and up to date. This is common sense advice. You shouldn't need the possibility of a pandemic to spur you into basic preparations that can keep you and your family safe—at any time.

TREATMENT FOR THE SEASONAL FLU— LESSONS TO BE LEARNED

The seasonality of influenza is one of the more intriguing aspects of non-pandemic flu. (At least it is to infectious disease specialists!)

The incidence of annual global influenza tends to spike twice each year, corresponding to the winter seasons in the northern and southern hemispheres. The best explanation for this spike in cases during the coldest months of the year is that people tend to remain indoors, in poorly ventilated rooms, and in close proximity to large numbers of people.

How contagious is the flu? How can I stop its spread?

The flu virus is extremely contagious. It can remain infectious on telephones and other surfaces for quite some time. Not hours, but *days.* Touching a contaminated surface may lead to infection as well. Whether at work or at home, **surfaces shared by others, such as desks, counter-tops, computer keypads, and telephones, should be disinfected at the start of, and the end of each day.** Use either Lysol, household bleach, or similar products.

In addition to getting the influenza vaccine, the prevention of seasonal flu requires fastidious personal hygiene. Avoiding contamination by the secretions of an infected individual require frequent hand cleansing. A good rule of thumb is to **vigorously wash your hands with soap and water for at least thirty seconds every two to three hours during flu season.** Soaps, by definition, dissolve lipid-bearing components of the viral surface. This disrupts the virus and makes it noninfectious. The brand isn't critical—even a mild soap such as Ivory works well. (Antibacterial soaps are more active against certain bacteria and spores.) When this is not practical, cleanse your hands with the same frequency by using an alcohol-based hand sanitizer, such as Purell.

Avoid close contact with obviously ill persons—with a radius of about six feet. In households, anyone who has upper respiratory congestion, nasal discharge, and/or runny eyes should sleep in separate beds from those who are not ill. Hugging, kissing, and other intimate contact should be deferred until the period of contagion is over. If it is necessary to care for a family member with the flu, a face mask and eye protection (such as Johnson & Johnson Barrier Protective Goggles or Centurion Splash Goggles) (see below) will certainly reduce the risk of infection. The household patient should spend most of their time in his or her own space or room. An adequate supply of hand disinfectant, tissues (not cloth handkerchiefs), and a closed container for used tissues should be readily accessible.

The most infectious particles are those that remain suspended in the air for long periods of time. These particles are usually in the range of 20 microns in diameter, and if inhaled by a healthy person, can reach the lower depths of the lung. Many people like to use humidifiers or steam vaporizers to add moisture to the air in the sickroom, thereby improving comfort to the dry mucous membranes of the upper respiratory tract. However, by adding small water droplets in the air, they may provide aerosol carriers for more efficient spreading of the influenza virus. Generally speaking, humidifiers are not recommended.

Instead, **there may be added protection by having an air purifier with a HEPA (High Efficiency Particulate Air Filtration) air filter,** or an ionic filter capable of trapping these circulating infectious particles. (Of course, when cleaning these devices—which should be done every few days—a face mask and eye protection is important.)

When you have the flu, one of the most dangerous things you can do is try to tough it out. No matter how pressing your tasks, you should *not* go to work for five to six days after the onset of flu symptoms. Most large employers have become very aware of workplace contamination, and have adopted lenient policies regarding sick leave during flu season. If you are ill with the flu, and you must leave your home for a doctor's visit or to run essential errands, a face mask is particularly useful in reducing the risk to those around you. While it may cause embarrassment, you should take solace in knowing that you are acting in a responsible and community-minded manner.

If you've gotten a seasonal flu shot, after about two weeks you *should* have antibodies to the current strains of the virus, and your body will be able to destroy the viral particles before they have a chance to invade your host cells and replicate. Otherwise, it can take anywhere from one to two weeks for your body to mount an effective immune response to the flu. However, there have been rare instances in which the designers of the seasonal flu vaccine have guessed wrong as to which strain to include in a particular year's inoculation. (In 2002, the Fujian strain of H1N2 influenza virus eluded the vaccine used that year.) Therefore, it's not wise to assume that your vaccine will provide infallible protection. Continue to use the personal protection measures described above.

Fortunately, we are not yet dealing with a human bird flu pandemic. What we know of the H5N1 infection in poultry, and in the few people infected thus far, is that the amount of virus shed is increased compared with the virus shed during the seasonal illness we are accustomed to. In addition, a person sick with bird flu is likely to have no partial acquired immunity, and will remain infectious for longer periods of time. The protective measures I've just discussed will become even more crucial in preventing the transmission of bird flu, should it arrive at our doorsteps.

ABOUT FACE MASKS

If there is a flu epidemic or pandemic and you still need to go outside, the best protection you'll have is with a properly fitting face mask.

The regular use of face masks is far more commonplace in certain cities in Asia, such as Tokyo in Japan or Ho Chi Minh City in Vietnam, where most Vespa riders in that crowded, polluted city cover their faces as soon as they hop on their scooters to go to work. Most Americans, however, would either chastise or shy away from anyone wearing a face mask in the subway, thinking that the masked person has either got something that he or she doesn't want to spread—or that they certainly don't want to catch. During an epidemic or pandemic, though, it's likely that the use of masks would be made mandatory, and their proliferation would be welcomed, not shunned.

You should also take care to cover your eyes with wraparound glasses or goggles, as well, as the influenza virus can eater the body through the tear ducts.

The N95 face mask is the industry standard. It can be quite uncomfortable to wear any mask if you have the flu and are having trouble breathing, or have a high fever that's making you feel extremely hot. But as masks might help reduce the risk of transmission from the sick person to the caregiver, risk reduction is more important than the comfort factor.

It's important to make sure an N95 mask fits correctly and has a tight seal on the skin, or wearing one will provide no protection. They are available in three different sizes, with the smallest fitting children.

The effectiveness of face masks depends on a proper fit. The material of the mask must filter all inhaled air into the nose and mouth—which means that absolutely no air gets in through the space between the mask and the skin of the face. Beards and moustaches pose special problems here, so they should be shaved off.

Proper fit testing of respirator masks is done by inhaling atomized saccharine (like Sweet and Low) in an enclosed space. Dissolve it in some water, put it in a spray bottle, then place the mask on. Spray the solution. If you can taste the sweetener, your mask is not secure. Regular sugar has no odor and won't work for this purpose.

Another method that is a bit more practical for home use is to put the mask on, then inhale briskly with your mouth opened. Watch yourself in the mirror as you do so. A proper fit will cause the mask to compress, or deflate, upon deep inhalation.

In addition, the new Nano Mask is also being touted as the first kind of face mask to use a filter media to isolate and destroy viral and bacterial pathogens. I suggest you research the different types of masks on the Internet, and order some to have on hand—most are not available in drugstores—just in case anyone in your family comes down with the seasonal flu, or any other respiratory illness.

How can I recognize influenza?

Rapid recognition of a case of influenza within a household is the first step toward preventing everyone else from developing secondary cases. Influenza may mimic many other infectious diseases. Hundreds of other viruses (rhinoviruses, echoviruses, enteroviruses, and so forth) can cause common cold-like symptoms.

In all human viral respiratory infections, the infectious period begins one to two days *before* the onset of symptoms, and lasts for upwards of a week after they appear. Which is why I recommended that you stay home from work for five to six days after becoming ill.

Influenza tends to cause a more severe illness than the common cold viruses. The flu usually makes its unwelcome appearance quite quickly. There can be a rapid onset of high fever (102 to 104 degrees), severe body and muscle aches, chills, prostration and weakness, headache, cough, shortness of breath, runny nose, and/or sore throat. You'll likely have little appetite, and be too exhausted to do anything except stay in bed from anywhere from two days to two weeks. The flu doesn't go away as quickly as it first appears, unfortunately, Although you can feel quite ill for a while, I reassure my patients that in the scope of all illnesses, they're not usually *that* sick.

As you read in chapter 1, 36,000 people in the United States alone die from seasonal influenza. How can a nonmedical person decipher who will recover on his or her own, and who needs immediate medical attention? Fortunately, there are warning signs.

First, remember that influenza kills mainly by impairing the body's ability to exchange oxygen from the air with carbon dioxide in the blood.

The lungs are the organs that achieve this function, so the dread signs of severe influenza relate to respiratory failure.

The normal number of breaths is twelve to sixteen per minute. A rapid breathing rate, called tachypnea, may be much higher, with twenty-five to forty breaths per minute. This indicates that the brain is sensing a need for more oxygen, and is signaling the body to breathe faster. Be aware that tachypnea also occurs when the body is stressed from such things as high temperature, so be sure to check the respiratory rate when the temperature has been reduced to normal.

Another way the body has to cope with early respiratory failure is to breathe more deeply, which is called hyperpnea. You probably have experienced the feeling of deep, gulping breaths after vigorous exercise. By increasing the volume of air exchanged with each breath, the body is able to oxygenate the blood more efficiently. A person in the early stages of respiratory failure will be using muscles other than the diaphragm to help with the breathing process, so the accessory respiratory muscles of the neck and the abdomen will be called into action. This is called "pulling" in the vernacular. A person struggling to exchange air will be using the neck muscles to tug on the collarbones and upper ribs, and the upper abdominal muscles to pull down on the lower ribs, thereby creating a bellows action on the chest wall. Such sustained use of accessory respiratory muscles is a critical warning sign of impending respiratory failure.

Your sense of hearing and touch may also give you information. Bubbling or crunching sounds of the chest, wheezing, or tactile vibrations during an intake of breath are signs that fluid is accumulating in the lung tissue. At the later stage of respiratory failure, when oxygen levels fall, heliotrope cyanosis develops. This is a blue or purplish hue, seen earliest in the nail beds and around the lips, but later all over the face and body. Urgent medical attention in an emergency room is indicated as soon as any of these signs or symptoms appear.

High temperature is a primitive innate immune response to infection of all types. While fever itself is seldom dangerous, temperatures in adults over 106 degrees can damage essential proteins and enzymes and disrupt normal biological functions. Monitoring of temperature is best accomplished rectally, or with the use of a digital ear probe. Oral thermometers may underestimate the temperature in anyone who is breathing rapidly and unable to keep his or her mouth comfortably closed for several minutes. Antipyretics, such as aspirin, Tylenol, or Advil-like medications are helpful in bringing the temperature down. (Note that aspirin is contraindicated in children because of the possibility of a serious complication called Reye's syndrome.)

The body also controls the fever by inducing sweating. The evaporation of sweat removes body heat. Sweating, as you know, requires the excretion of water from the sweat glands of the skin. Hence, dehydration will interfere with the body's ability to lower the temperature. Avoid piling on blankets and clothing in a patient who feels chilled because of the effects of sweating. This will only maintain a high body temperature. A light sheet should be used instead.

A seriously ill person will lose excessive amounts of fluid—up to one liter for every degree of elevation of body temperature. Fluids are also lost through respiration, especially in patients breathing at excessive rates. Dehydration is a very serious complication of influenza. As the blood volume diminishes due to lost fluids, the blood pressure will begin to fall. To preserve adequate blood flow to the vital organs, such as the brain and the heart, blood vessels to other organs close down. Kidney and liver failure then ensue, and shock and death is not far behind.

The signs of dehydration are easy to detect. Patients will stop sweating. The mucous membranes of the mouth feel bone dry, and the skin loses its resilience. A good test for dehydration is to pinch the skin of the top of the hand and pull it up gently. If it remains "tented," the patient is probably very dehydrated. The abdominal wall may also become "tented" or doughy in texture.

What is the best medical treatment for influenza?

I've just discussed some of the warning signs that should alert you to seek immediate medical attention for anyone with influenza. Remember that if you become ill with influenza, medical treatment may reduce the severity of your disease—and may even save your life. Even if your condition, or that of your family member, is not critical, medical treatment may lessen your illness and get you on the road to recovery more rapidly.

Over-the-counter medications such as decongestants may help reduce discomfort, help you sleep, and as stated above, lessen contagiousness. Do remember that over-the-counter products expire, so don't plan on downing the cough syrup you'd stashed in the closet the last time you had the flu without checking the label. There have been examples where certain products have actually become dangerously degraded past their expiration date.

Sometimes, annoying symptoms such as a runny nose or cough can persist for weeks after the initial infection. If they're viral in nature, they can't be treated with antibiotics. If they are secondary bacterial infections—such as bacterial pneumonia, bronchitis, sinus infections, or ear infections (especially in young children)—you may be prescribed antibiotics by your health care provider. Those with chronic medical conditions, such as congestive heart failure, asthma, or diabetes, may be more prone to the bacterial complications of influenza.

FDA-approved anti-viral medications that have been shown to reduce the intensity and duration of influenza are covered in chapter 8. If you are prescribed Tamiflu, or one of the other available drugs, it is best taken upon the first appearance of any flu symptoms, and for five subsequent days.

How can the flu virus be destroyed outside the body?

Influenza virus is destroyed by heat ($167-212°F$ [$75-100°C$]). It's also inactivated by chemical germicides such as chlorine bleach, hydrogen peroxide, detergents (soap), iodine-based antiseptics, and alcohol. Clorox bleach and Lysol disinfectant are viricides.

You can also vigilantly use alcohol-based hand sanitizers, such as Purell or Microsan, when going out in public, as well as at work. You'd be amazed at the amount of pathogens lurking on seemingly clean surfaces. Taxicabs, doorknobs, subways and buses, pay phones, and restrooms can be filthy. So is paper money. Try to get in the habit of keeping a small bottle of hand sanitizer available for use at all times, especially for wiping down surfaces in your office.

Washing your hands can also save your life. This doesn't mean you should use a dab of soap and be done with it—the mechanical action, more than hot water or detergent, is what's crucial. The action of washing your hands reduces the amount of infectious agents, bacteria, and viruses. Soap also inactivates the surface membranes of certain germs as well.

FOOD PREPARATION TIPS

As H5N1 has infected and killed millions of chickens, ducks, turkeys, and geese, it is quite logical to wonder if there is any danger within our food supply.

Fortunately, Low Pathogen Avian Influenza (LPAI) in birds, the viral type most commonly found in America, is not transmissible by eating poultry.

During a recent government briefing, Dr. Richard Raymond, the under secretary for Food Safety at the United States Department of Agriculture (USDA) spoke about what is worrisome, and what is not. Theoretically, he admitted, we need to be concerned about eating raw poultry products from diseased birds, especially as there have been documented cases in Vietnam of people becoming ill with bird flu after eating dishes prepared with raw duck blood (as I detailed in chapter 3).

"If High Pathogen Avian Influenza (HPAI) were to be detected in the United States, I want to assure the American public that the chance of that infected poultry ever entering the food chain would be extremely low," Dr. Raymond said. "That's in part because we have inspection personnel from the USDA's Food Safety and Inspection Service assigned to every federally inspected meat, poultry, and egg product plant in America. Poultry products for public consumption are inspected for signs of disease both before and after slaughter. The 'inspected for wholesomeness by the U.S. Department of Agriculture' seal ensures that this poultry is free from visible signs of disease.

"No human cases of avian influenza have been confirmed from eating properly prepared poultry," he added. "In addition to proper processing in the plants, proper handling and cooking of poultry also provides protection from viruses and bacteria including the avian influenza.

"But I want to reiterate at this point that proper food safety practices are important every day. As an agency we remind consumers each day and every day that there are basic food safety steps to follow. That's clean, separate, cook, and chill.

"By clean we mean always wash your hands and surfaces that have come in contact with meat and poultry products before and after handling food.

"By separate we mean don't cross-contaminate. Keep raw meat, poultry, fish, and their juices away from other foods. Cooking a turkey breast at an adequate temperature does no good if you've contaminated the lettuce. Cooking the meat and poultry to the proper temperatures using the food thermometer is the only sure way to know that you have cooked that product properly. Appearance will not answer that question for you.

"A high enough temperature will destroy bacteria and viruses in poultry products. The USDA specifically recommends cooking ground turkey and ground chicken to a temperature of 165 degrees Fahrenheit; cook turkey breast to 170 degrees Fahrenheit; and whole birds, legs, thighs, and wings to 185 degrees Fahrenheit.

"And then chill. Refrigerate promptly. Always refrigerate perishable foods within two hours of taking it out of the refrigerator or having prepared it by proper cooking. And as a reminder, refrigerators should be at 40 degrees Fahrenheit or lower, and freezers should be at zero degrees Fahrenheit or lower."

In addition, you should cook all eggs thoroughly. Wash eggshells in soapy water before handling and cooking, and wash your hands afterward. Egg yolks should not be runny or liquid, and never consumed raw. If you're baking and use raw eggs, don't be tempted to taste the batter!

No one in any country in the world should now be tempted to eat any dish containing uncooked flesh or blood from any bird.

Sanitize cutting boards and countertops with a solution of one teaspoon of chlorine bleach per quart of water.

PREPARATION FOR A PANDEMIC

In chapter 6, I outlined the global strategies currently in place to monitor the progress of H5N1 outbreaks—in the bird population, and in the human population. Now let's talk about what you can do right now.

What can I do to get ready for a pandemic?

Aside from getting your house in order and stockpiling supplies, in truth, there's very little you can actually *physically* do if there is a pandemic. (Of course, you've already gotten your seasonal flu shot, right?)

Emotionally, on the other hand, you can stave off worries by educating yourself about how to treat the flu to minimize its spread; accept the fact that life as you know it will be severely curtailed during a pandemic; and stay informed about H5N1's spread in birds by reading reputable news reports. (Use the Resources section to find helpful links.)

As I discussed in chapter 6, there is already a global surveillance system, however imperfect, in place to keep a wary eye on H5N1 infections. Should the virus mutate, it will probably not be like a *War of the Worlds* alien invasion springing seemingly out of nowhere to scare us to death. There *will* be some warning.

We learned many lessons after the SARS scare in 2003. Right from the beginning, that virus had the ability to jump from person to person much the same way that the flu is spread—by respiratory secretions (coughing and sneezing). The health-care workers tending to patients quickly sickened, and many of them died.

This is unlikely to happen with H5N1. If it mutates, it's likely to hit one person here, and another person there, before clusters begin to emerge. If a pandemic is indeed starting to unfold, we'll first go through WHO Stage 5 (new virus causes human cases, with evidence of significant human-to-human transmission) before we hit Stage 6, a full-blown pandemic with efficient and sustained human-to-human transmission. Remember, H5N1 has been percolating in the bird population in Asia for at least the past seven years, and it still has *not* been able to make that next deadly step.

In the meantime, what you can do is maximize your health to minimize your risk for all contagious illnesses. This means keeping keep yourself as healthy as possible: maintaining a healthy weight, exercising regularly, curbing any bad habits such as excessive drinking or smoking, getting a good night's rest, minimizing stress levels, educating yourself about bird flu—which means maintaining a healthy skepticism about what bloggers are saying about the bird flu.

You can also use this as an opportunity to have a talk with your primary care physician, especially if you've made an appointment to get that crucial seasonal flu shot. Before your appointment, go to the reputable websites listed in the Resources section and carefully read the information therein, or bring in a copy of this book. See what your physician suggests, and if he or she is connected to infectious disease specialists should the need arise. Ask if you might be a candidate for the pneumococcal vaccine, a shot that can help prevent pneumonia and is recommended for seniors and those at higher risk for respiratory ailments. (The pneumococcal vaccine is routinely given to nearly all infants, has few side effects, and remains effective for five to ten years, longer if a booster is given.) If an epidemic or pandemic seems to be closer to reality, it might be a good time to ask for a prescription for a standard antibiotic that can treat the secondary bacterial infections that can arise after a bout with the viral flu. (Never, of course, self-diagnose or take any antibiotics without specific instructions from your doctor.) During a pandemic, when movement is severely curtailed, it obviously may not be possible to have any prescriptions filled.

It is also a good idea to have a family emergency plan in place—for any emergency situation. If a parent is at work, or there are children in school, when a pandemic alert is announced, how will everyone connect? Where is the family meeting place? Who is the backup care provider? How will everyone be reached? One of the lessons learned on 9/11 was that cell phone networks are vulnerable during disasters. Always keep a working landline phone that is not dependent on the main electricity grid on hand, just in case.

Do you think people will be compliant with instructions from public health officials if there is a pandemic?

I certainly hope so, although it's hard to predict how people will act during an overwhelming health crisis. If the experience of 1918 is repeated, most people will be so terrified of exposure to the flu that they will shut themselves inside, hoping not to become infected until the pandemic has passed. Our nation's largest cities became virtual ghost towns. But, back then, most people didn't have telephones and quick communication was next to impossible. That's certainly not the case now, unless of course the electricity fails when employees don't show up for work, and the utilities companies can't run at peak strength.

As a physician, I often must deal with recalcitrant patients who aren't compliant. Many do not perceive themselves as vulnerable, or they distrust traditional medical approaches to disease. They don't want to take their medications and they don't want to change their risky behavior.

The most valuable lesson I have learned in my twenty-four years of medical practice has been to view the patient as the critical half of a medical care team. I listen to my patients' concerns, respect their fears and opinions, but demand the same of them. I do not hesitate to express disappointment when they make bad or arbitrary decisions. If patients believe that their physicians have their best interests in mind, they are more likely to consider doing the right thing.

When it comes to flu pandemics, the patient, family members, and significant others will be doing most of the front-line triage and management. By taking the time to educate and instruct patients, physicians help them navigate a very frightening eventuality. It is also important for the physician to practice what he or she preaches. Many patients have asked me if I have had my flu shot (the answer is yes). Many, too, have asked if I have stockpiled Tamiflu for my own family (the answer is no). We are *all* facing the same risk and fears.

PANDEMIC PREPAREDNESS IN THE HOME

If there is a pandemic, chances are high that an attempt to impose a regional and/or national quarantine will be enacted for a short period of time. Open noncontained spaces obviously are going to be a lot safer than being in a small, closed office or room or house or wherever there are sick people around. People will be advised to stay at home (rather than evacuate, as they may be told to do before a natural disaster such as a hurricane), to lessen the possibility of exposure to those already infected or ill.

It may also take time for local officials to bring relief to areas overwhelmed by illness. Most likely, people will be reluctant to leave the house unless the need is dire. A high percentage of businesses would temporarily close or curtail their activities, as most of the workforce would either be ill, or caring for family members who may be.

For that reason, you should have essential supplies on hand. I suggest that you stock up on enough food and especially water for each family member, including pets, for at least a week. If you have the storage space (bottled water is bulky), store as much as you can. This is a smart move in general, as natural disasters, such as blizzards, floods, and hurricanes, can always strike, sometimes with little warning. Besides, stocking up on supplies is never a waste of money. Food and water stockpiled in the pantry can always be eaten and drunk when they're close to expiration dates, and replenished with fresh supplies.

The best source for information about disaster preparedness in the home is the Red Cross. They suggest the following basic supplies, with more detailed instructions at their website:

- *Water*: Human beings can live for many weeks without adequate food, especially if activities are reduced as they presumably would be during a quarantine period, but they can only survive a few days without water.

  Clean drinking water as well as water for hygiene and food preparation is a must during an emergency situation. A good estimate is to store a gallon of water per day for each healthy person and pet in your household. You can also fill up bathtubs with water should supplies of bottled water run low.

- *Food*: Store at least a three-day supply of nonperishable food that needs no refrigeration, preparation, or cooking. Ideal foods to store include canned juices; canned fruit and vegetables, especially beans and legumes; canned protein sources such as tuna, meats, and peanut butter; staples (sugar, salt, flour, spices); high energy foods, such as energy bars; enriched cereal; vitamins; and comfort/stress foods.

  Those with infants should have formula, powdered milk, bottles and nipples, and jars of baby food and snacks. In addition, you'll need a large supply of diapers and wipes.

Those with pets should have an adequate supply of canned/dry food.

Be sure to have a nonelectric can opener on hand.

• *First-aid supplies*: You should always have a first-aid kit in an easy-to-reach place. It should contain bandages, sterile dressings, gauze pads, germicidal wipes and hand sanitizer, nonlatex gloves, tape, antibacterial ointment, a cold pack, scissors, tweezers, a thermometer, and face masks.

Over-the-counter medications should include aspirin and nonaspirin pain relievers, cough syrup, anti-diarrhea medicines, antacids, dental needs, and contact lens supplies.

Anyone with a medical condition should have an adequate supply of their prescription medications on hand. Keep eyeglasses and sunglasses handy, too.

• *Tools and emergency supplies*: You'll need paper cups, plates, and plastic utensils; a battery-operated radio; lots and lots of assorted sizes of batteries; a working flashlight; cash; utility knives; a fire extinguisher; a basic tool kit; matches; plastic storage containers and plastic sheeting; needles and thread; toilet paper; wipes; soap; liquid detergent; personal hygiene items; disinfectant; household chlorine bleach; and tight-sealing plastic buckets.

• *Paperwork*: In addition to food and emergency supplies, you should also have your paperwork in order, filed in a lightweight container. Ideally, you should have originals of your will, insurance policies, contracts deeds, stocks and bonds, passports, social security cards, other ID cards, family records (birth, marriage, death certificates), tax returns, and immunization records. Write down all your bank account numbers, credit card account numbers, and contact information, as well as crucial telephone numbers. Storing them in your cell phone will be useless if it doesn't work any longer.

• *Pets*: Your beloved animals need to be taken care of as well. The Humane Society suggests at least a week's supply of food and water, pet medications, veterinary records, leashes or harnesses, and a current photo of your pet(s). Have plenty of plastic bags and newspapers as well as containers and cleaning supplies to help deal with pet waste. Puppy training pads are also useful for this purpose.

• *Entertainment*: Life will go on during a pandemic. Even during terrifying national disasters, those confined to the home may start to go stir-crazy. Have decks of cards, board games, good books, paper and pens/crayons/paint, and toys for the children in ample supply.

WILL WE BE QUARANTINED
IF A PANDEMIC BREAKS OUT?

In a discussion sponsored by the State Department, Dr. Karen Smith, public health director for Napa County, California, answered questions about H5N1. When asked about the possibility of a quarantine during a pandemic, she replied: "It isn't really possible to impose quarantine on a country. Quarantine generally refers to restrictions placed on the movements of people within an area that is affected by a disease.

"Quarantine can only be imposed by those with legal control over the area in question," she went on. "Thus the government of Country A can impose quarantine on certain of its citizens or even places within that country, but no other country could impose a quarantine on Country A. Country B could, however, refuse to import birds or allow people from Country A to enter Country B, but that would not be a quarantine.

"When quarantine is imposed on a person or area, the duration of that quarantine depends on the legal authority imposing the quarantine. In California, for example, quarantine would be imposed on someone who appears well (i.e., is not sick), but has been exposed to a communicable disease, and is within the incubation period of the disease. That person presents a risk to others with whom she/he comes into contact because she/he could develop the disease and spread it to those others. In this case, the person under quarantine can only be restricted until the incubation period of the disease has passed. At that point, if that person has not become sick, we know that she/he will not become sick and, therefore, no longer poses a risk to anyone else and quarantine must end. Our law is written so that the duration of quarantine depends on the disease in question. If it is not yet established, the duration of quarantine is determined by the local Public Health Officer but must be supported by science."

Given the population of our country, as well as in other countries, imposing a widespread quarantine is logistically impossible. I'd venture a guess that only those working in hospitals or other facilities where there are large clusters of sick people will be able to enact any kind of enforceable quarantine.

FLU PROTECTION WHILE TRAVELING

At the moment, the CDC has not recommended that travelers, both on business and for pleasure, avoid trips to any the countries where people have died from the H5N1 bird flu virus. So far, these countries are China, Vietnam, Cambodia, Thailand, and Indonesia.

Their recommendations are as follows (for more complete information, go to the CDC website):

Before you leave:
- Assemble a travel health kit containing basic first aid and medical supplies. Be sure to include a thermometer and alcohol-based hand rub for hand hygiene.
- Educate yourself and others who may be traveling with you about influenza.
- Be sure you are up to date with all recommended vaccinations, and see your health-care provider at least four to six weeks before travel to get any additional inoculations or information you may need.
- Check your health insurance plan or purchase additional insurance that covers medical evacuation in case you become sick and need to return home. You should not travel on a regular commercial airline if you are sick.
- Identify in-country health-care resources in advance of your trip.

While you are in an area where bird flu cases have been reported:
- Avoid areas with live poultry, such as live animal markets and poultry farms.
- Avoid places such as poultry farms and bird markets where live poultry are raised or kept, and avoid contact with sick or dead poultry. (Large amounts of the virus are known to be excreted in the droppings from infected birds.)
- As with other infectious illnesses, one of the most important and appropriate preventive practices is careful and frequent hand hygiene. Cleaning your hands often using either soap and water or waterless alcohol-based hand sanitizers removes potentially infectious materials from your skin and helps prevent disease transmission.

WHAT ABOUT MY PETS?

According to Dr. Teresa Telecky, former director of the Wildlife Trade Program at the Humane Society and currently a consultant there, now is not the time to be thinking about buying *any* kind of bird, as an isolated case of H5N1 could quickly infect a large population of other birds. Although the United States has banned all importation of all breeds of pet birds and poultry from countries infected with the H5N1 virus, and although a thirty-day quarantine is in place for all pet birds and poultry imported from other countries, the Humane Society believes that it's just not worth the potential risk at the moment. Birds smuggled into the country and sold to unethical pet store owners may be tainted without our knowledge.

In the meantime, here are some simple precautions to take to ensure the health and well-being of all your pets:

- If you already have pet birds, keep them isolated from *any* potential contact with wild birds. Keep all pet birds inside at all times; do not hang their cages on porches or other outdoor areas.
- As bird viruses are usually asymptomatic, this would be a good time to have a checkup with the vet and a simple blood test taken to look for any viruses.
- Keep your birds away from any other pet birds belonging to friends and neighbors, as well.
- Do not feed wild birds. Stay away from all wild birds. Never attempt to catch them or touch them.
- If you have animals, such as dogs or cats, who are allowed outside without a leash, do not let them go near any fields, or ponds or other bodies of water where wild birds may have landed or nested. It is especially crucial to prevent them digging near or swimming in any bodies of water where wild birds have landed, as the H5N1 virus is shed in the feces of wild birds.
- If any of your pets have had any contact with wild birds and then show symptoms of the flu, seek immediate medical attention from your veterinarian.

• Influenza viruses are destroyed by heat; therefore, as a precaution, all foods from poultry, including eggs, should be thoroughly cooked.
• If you develop respiratory symptoms or any illness that requires prompt medical attention, a U.S. consular officer can assist in locat-

ing appropriate medical services and informing family or friends.
• It is advisable that you do not travel until you are free of symptoms.

After your return:
• Monitor your health for ten days.
• If you become ill with fever or respiratory symptoms during this ten-day period, consult a health-care provider. Before your visit to a health-care setting, tell the provider about your symptoms and recent travel so that he or she can be aware you have traveled to an area reporting avian influenza.

Chapter 10.

CONCLUSION: IT'S NOT IF, BUT *WHEN* (and *HOW BAD*)

Men believe only that it is a divine disease because of their
ignorance and amazement.

—*Hippocrates*

It is a fair assumption that people and birds have exchanged strains of viral pathogens for millennia. Pandemics have been recorded in the history books for hundreds of years. Without question, another people/bird pandemic will surface again at some time in the future.

But, with so many factors currently involved, we just can't predict with any certainty whether an H5N1 pandemic is about to unfold now.

Or when.

At a meeting at the New York University School of Medicine on November 28, 2005, Dr. Jeffery Taubenberger, one of the decoders of the 1918 pandemic flu genome and a thought-leader in the science of human influenza, spoke to a large and rapt audience of researchers and clinicians. Dr. Taubenberger's work on the genome was published in the prestigious publications *Science* and *Nature* in October 2005. During the question-and-answer period, he was asked to predict whether the H5N1 avian virus would jump to humans.

His response was: "I am on the fence with that answer."

Even a brilliant scientist, who lives and breathes influenza, could not reach a solid prediction based on the information and evidence in hand.

If *he* can't, how can *you*?

From my experience, I'd say that many people, including most of my patients, tend to express two diametrically opposed sentiments about the bird flu right now.

The first comes from patients who've read about H5N1, and are concerned and anxious, but do not know really how to prepare for the eventuality of another pandemic. "Can I have some Tamiflu?" they ask.

The second comes from patients that prefer the more cavalier approach to life's problems. "So what if there are a lot of birds flying around right now that might end up killing us—*I just don't want to think about it*," they say.

In order to take action, you first must admit there is a problem. And there's no getting around the fact that H5N1 is a problem. Right now, it's a devastating problem for the bird population in Asia. It's been devastating for the friends and loved ones of the seventy-four people who've died from it.

But H5N1 is not *yet* a globally devastating problem. As I said in the last chapter, this virus has had seven years in which it could have mutated into a form transmissible easily from person to person, but it didn't. Maybe this virus never will cause a human pandemic. Yet in the context of revisiting the 1918 H1N1 pandemic, even if that was the worst-case scenario, we need to accept the possibility that this, or some other avian influenza virus, will again cause mass human suffering and death.

Viruses mutate—that's what they do. In fact, a rather alarming report out of China's Xinhua news agency at the end of November 2005 claimed that the H5N1 strain of bird flu detected in human cases there has mutated when compared with strains found in human cases in Vietnam. We've got to be prepared as H5N1, and all avian flu strains, continue to mutate.

As you know by now, the problem is viral unpredictability. As such, they're like natural disasters. In California, we know which fault lines run near which big cities, and we can track seismic activity with great accuracy. We know how often these fault lines have shifted in the past. We can read about statistical probabilities and likelihood of a disaster. But seismologists can't predict when the next Big One will rattle San Francisco or Los Angeles. A Big One in California *will* happen at some point in the future; it can't *not,* as the geological pressure is simply too intense to contain it.

The next avian flu pandemic will give us some warning signs well in advance of the first wave. We have already had a seven-year period in which to study the properties of H5N1. Hopefully, if H5N1 is our next pandemic, it will give us further time to perform pathogen surveillance in the bird population, and to develop strategies for prevention and treatment of humans who become infected. I am very hopeful that the genomic projects now underway (discussed in chapter 8) will provide the basis for understanding the precise molecular mechanisms by which the virus can shift its target host from bird to human. And while the scientific community works on this problem, I believe that the methods being used to stem the extent of bird infection will buy them more time to realize significant breakthroughs that will translate into effective treatment and prevention strategies.

I think it's instructive to look back at the early days of the AIDS epidemic, when it was a horrendous disease that seemed to have sprung out of nowhere to kill off the gay community. People usually died within seven to eight months of being diagnosed. I was asked to consult for some large corporations that were trying to conduct business as usual. They feared that if one of their employees were diagnosed with AIDS, the whole office would come to a crashing halt. No one would use the telephones or the bathrooms. People wouldn't come to work until the place was fumigated. And in fact, one of my patients actually received a "pink-slip" with the notation "effective immediately" the day after he was admitted to the hospital for pneumonia. Clearly, ignorance about the mode of spread of AIDS fueled the over-the-top anxiety and reaction to the disease.

Until we learned how the virus was transmitted, and how to begin to treat it, there was plenty of hysteria. Although over a million Americans have been infected, 500,000 have died, and an estimated 40,000 new HIV infections occur in the United States every year, what was once a horrendous disease has become a manageable disease, where those infected with

HIV can live a normal life span. *Nobody* back in 1982 would have predicted that we would be where we are today, with a healthy infected population. I certainly wouldn't have.

Which brings me to the take-home message about bird flu. Our *best* ultimate protection against this deadly disease will come not through public information programs, government policies, grass-roots interventions to change poultry raising methods, or even from the pharmaceutical industry—it will derive from raw science. To get technical about it: Laboratory research using all of the modern molecular biology marvels will dissect the precise mutation patterns that correlate with human infectivity, pathogenicity, and transmission. Then the translational sciences will use those basic science breakthroughs, and convert them into testable treatments, preventative vaccines, and diagnostic tests.

In other words, scientists doing dogged, determined, relentless work will figure out how specific viruses mutate. When they do, we'll be able to effectively treat them in a timely manner.

Imagine a laboratory able to detect an influenza A gene segment that's common to all bird flu strains, one that makes it critical to the infectivity of all the bird flu strains. If such a gene is discovered, theoretically, a "super vaccine" could be developed. This super vaccine might then prevent against *all* strains of the flu, regardless of minor mutations. As a result, the world's population could be vaccinated against bird flu, eradicating it from the human population. Can you imagine the relief there'd be if we no longer had to suffer from the flu?

A super vaccine for the flu *is* a possibility, much as smallpox and polio vaccine programs have wiped most of those diseases off the globe. Scientific progress should always remain the basis of our optimism. And we should invest richly in promising research programs.

In many ways, medical science has set the stage for the current obsession over bird flu, pandemics, and infectious diseases in general. Childhood vaccination programs have prevented a wide array of infectious diseases, decreased child mortality, and increased life expectancy in developed countries. Childbirth is no longer so risky for either mother and baby. Antibiotics treat the routine infections that follow surgical procedures.

As a result, the general public has come to expect treatments, prevention, and cures for many of the previously insoluble conditions that sickened and killed prior generations. We've also come to expect that we're not going to die of disease. Which is why so many people are seriously displeased (if not enraged) when they have a virus and they can't take a pill to make it go away.

Disease is, after all, extremely inconvenient.

So is complacency. International travel, the information age, and threat of biological terrorism have reduced the comforting insulation we've grown accustomed to in this country. With reams of information available in virtual real-time, average citizens, already shaken by 9/11, Anthrax, threats of bioterrorism, and discussions of smallpox resurgence, have justifiably reacted with concern, anxiety, and fear.

Even, at times, with pandemic panic.

And with the White House elevating the possibility of an influenza epidemic to an issue impacting national security, all bets are off. Or are they?

I'd lay off the betting for now. When I was much younger, I was a rather intense young man, and I took many of the problems of the day to heart, more than most of my peers. After hearing me express some of these concerns and fears—okay, I *was* ranting a bit—my wise uncle would always ask, "What were you worried about five years ago?" He stopped me in my tracks, as I never could recall those worries.

In other words, *this too shall pass.*

Which brings me back to what I said at the beginning of this chapter: Without question, another people/bird pandemic will surface again. If our country's preparations work, we'll have moved science forward in much-needed ways. "First, we'll have cell-based technology that will allow us the capacity to produce vaccines in sufficient size and within the constraints of time," said HHS secretary Michael Leavitt. "Second, we will have made substantial progress in expanding our annual flu capacity. Third, we will have better state and local preparedness for any medical emergency. Fourth, we'll have an international network of disease surveillance that will serve this country and others. And last, we'll have peace of mind of knowing we're ready."

Let's hope that we will indeed be ready. And that the knowledge we acquire today will help us confront the infectious disease threats of tomorrow.

ACKNOWLEDGMENTS

My career in infectious diseases has been an ongoing journey that has allowed me the privilege of observing how the human spirit, hopefulness, and perseverance can prevail over microbes. To my thousands of patients, please know that a deeper gratitude could never be felt.

Dr. Saul J. Farber, the former dean provost and chairman of medicine at the New York University School of Medicine was, and continues to be, a true mentor and role model for me. I credit him with teaching me, and so many others, that the basis for good medicine is hard work, a love of science, and above all respect for the patient. The image of him examining a patient flashes before me every time I reach for my stethoscope.

And to my loving family: my wife, Miriam, and daughters, Ariel and Emily, for knowing that they were not second when it seemed I put my career first.

RESOURCES

Online Resources

Government and UN Organizations

Centers for Disease Control and Prevention (CDC)
www.cdc.gov/flu/avian/gen-info. Gives key facts about avian influenza, previous
international flu pandemics, avian infections in humans, transmission between
animals and people, spread among birds, and comparisons between various
types of flu and avian flu viruses.

European Union (EU)
http://europa.eu.int/comm/dgs/health_consumer/dyna/influenza/index.cfm.
Includes various fact sheets of frequently asked questions and continually updated press releases.

Food and Agriculture Organization of the United Nations (FAO)
http://www.fao.org/ag/againfo/home/en/home.html. Links to Animal Production and Health Division of the FAO's agriculture department. Features links to a
time line and maps of world outbreaks, along with other extensive resources.

Link to FAO: http://www.fao.org/ag/againfo/subjects/en/health/diseases-cards/avian_qa.html.

Food and Drug Administration (FDA)
http://www.fda.gov/cdrh/emergency/flu_qa.html. Fact sheet on using personal protective equipment (specialized gear) during influenza outbreaks.

Medline Plus (a collaborative research service of the U.S. National Library of Medicine and the National Institutes of Health)
http://www.nlm.nih.gov/medlineplus/birdflu.html. Links to dozen of recent news articles, fact sheets, and clinical trial details. Can also search Medline Plus for more specific articles.

National Wildlife Health Center (United States Geological Survey)
http://www.nwhc.usgs.gov/research/avian_influenza/avian_influenza.html. Basic information, news updates, health bulletins, maps, and resources relating to avian influenza.

Pandemicflu.gov
The official U.S. government website for information on pandemic flu and avian influenza.

U.S. Department of Health and Human Services
http://www.hhs.gov/pandemicflu/plan/. Allows visitors to download various documents relating to preparedness and response, including the entire 396-page plan, an eighteen-page overview, and specialized plans for various agencies (e.g., hospitals, school systems, local governments).

U.S. Department of State
http://usinfo.state.gov/gi/global_issues/bird_flu.html. Official documents, resources, and news about bird flu, including downloadable publication "Meeting the Challenge of Bird Flu." Travel Recommendations from USDS: http://travel.state.gov/travel/tips/health/health_2747.html.

USDA
http://www.usda.gov/wps/portal/!ut/p/_s.7_0_A/7_0_1OB?navid=AVIAN INFLUENZA&navtype=SU. Features frequently updated fact sheets, print news, webcasts, transcripts of official briefings, and more.

The White House
http://www.whitehouse.gov/homeland/pandemic-influenza.html. Comprehensive information about U.S. national strategy in combating pandemic influenza. Includes letter from President, historical information, the U.S. government's plans, and roles and responsibilities of government at all levels. Also: http://www.whitehouse.gov/news/releases/2005/11/20051101.html. November 1 outline of President's plan to safeguarding America against pandemic influenza. (At present, http://www.whitehouse.gov/infocus/healthcare/ links to information about bird flu as well.)

World Health Organization (WHO)
http://www.who.int/en/. The World Health Organization (UN's specialized agency for health). The right-hand side of the home page provides links on the current situation.

Disaster Preparedness

National Center for Disaster Preparedness
http://www.ncdp.mailman.columbia.edu/. The NCDP is an academically based resource center dedicated to the study, analysis, and enhancement of the nation's ability to prepare for and respond to major disasters, including terrorism. No specific information on bird flu.

Red Cross
www.redcross.org. Can search for news and press releases relating to avian influenza. Has a link on home page to pandemicflu.gov but otherwise, provides no Red Cross–specific data on bird flu.

Scientific Organizations

Center for Infectious Disease Research & Policy (CIDRAP), University of Minnesota
http://www.cidrap.umn.edu/cidrap/content/influenza/avianflu/index.html. Comprehensive resource for general information, updated news articles, journal articles, and links to governmental and other sites.

Infectious Diseases Society of America (IDSA)
http://www.idsociety.org. The IDSA represents physicians, scientists, and other health care professionals who specialize in infectious diseases. IDSA's purpose is

to improve the health of individuals, communities, and society by promoting excellence in patient care, education, research, public health, and prevention relating to infectious diseases. Can search for flu-related information and commentary.

International Society of Infectious Diseases
http://www.promedmail.org/pls/promed/f?p=2400:1000. Provides latest news about spread of avian influenza around the world, emergency medicine.

Mayo Clinic
http://www.mayoclinic.com/health/bird-flu/DS00566. Gives practical information on bird flu including historical overview, signs and symptoms, causes, risk factors, treatment, and prevention.

Daily English Newspapers for Asian/Pacific Countries

Australia
The *Melbourne Age*: www.theage.com.au

Cambodia
Phnom Penh Post: http://phnompenhpost.com/

China
South China Morning Post: http://www.scmp.com/

Hong Kong
Asia Times: http://www.atimes.com/

India
The *Indian Express*: http://www.indianexpress.com/
The *Times of India*: lhttp://timesofindia.indiatimes.com/

Indonesia
The *Jakarta Post*: www.thejakartapost.com

Japan
The *Japan Times*: http://www.japantimes.co.jp/
Asahi Shimbun: http://www.asahi.com/english/index.html (very basic)

Korea
The *Korea Herald*: http://www.koreaherald.co.kr/index.asp
The *Korea Times*: http://times.hankooki.com/

Malaysia
Malaysia Kini: http://www.malaysiakini.com/
The *Star Online*: http://biz.thestar.com.my/

The Maldives
Maldives Globe: http://www.maldivesglobe.com

Philippines
Philippine Star: http://www.philstar.com
The *Manila Times*: http://www.manilatimes.net/

Taiwan
The *China Post*: www.chinapost.com.tw
The *Taipei Times*: http://www.taipeitimes.com

Thailand
The *Bangkok Post*: http://www.bangkokpost.net
The Nation: http://www.nationmultimedia.com/2005/12/01/

Singapore
The *Straits Times*: http://straitstimes.asia1.com.sg
Also: Bird flu information site of the Singapore government: http://www.flu
.gov.sg/. Comprehensive site.

Vietnam
The *Vietnam Chronicle*: http://www.vietnamchronicle.com/

Africa
http://allafrica.com/stories/200511300376.html. AllAfrica.com, news site. (This
specific link, for instance, is a bird flu story from *Ethiopian Herald* about the
WHO declaring that Ethiopia is at greater risk for the bird flu, 11/30/05.)

Other News Sources

BBC's bird flu coverage
http://news.bbc.co.uk/1/hi/in_depth/world/2005/bird_flu/default.stm.

Bird Flu Today
http://www.birdflutoday.com/. Latest news from the World News (WN) Network (from wire and other official media outlets).

iFlu.org
http://www.ifu.org/. News and commentary on pandemic flu posted chronologically, supplied largely from Yahoo! News.

NPR
http://www.npr.org/templates/story/story.php?storyId=4949542&sourceCode=gaw. Links to all bird-flu related radio pieces, FAQ, and online resources.

UK NewsNow
http://newsnow.co.uk/newsfeed/?feed/?name=Bird+Flu. Monitors breaking news in fifteen languages from thousands of the Internet's most important online publications. (Site uses country flag icons to indicate source of news item; good way of seeing where information is coming from.)

Yahoo! News Bird Flu

http://news.search.yahoo.com/search/news?p=intitle%3Abird+intitle%3Aflu&ei=UTF-8. Articles culled from mainstream media outlets.

Publications

BMC Infectious Diseases
http://www.biomedcentral.com/bmcinfectdis/. Publishes original research articles in all aspects of the prevention, diagnosis, and management of infectious and sexually transmitted diseases, as well as related molecular genetics, pathophysiology, and epidemiology. *BMC Infectious Diseases* (ISSN 1471-2334) is indexed/tracked/covered by PubMed, MEDLINE, CAS, Scopus, EMBASE, ISI, and Google Scholar. Free registration required.

Bulletin of the World Health Organization—An International Journal of Public Health
http://www.who.int/bulletin/en/

Far Eastern Economic Review
http://www.feer.com/

Health Promotion International
http://heapro.oxfordjournals.org. An Official Journal of the International Union for Health Promotion and Education; published quarterly in association with the World Health Organization.

International Journal of Infectious Diseases
Indexed (searchable) on Medline. http://www.isid.org/publications/ijid.shtml (can't view content, only a description of the journal.)

Journal of the American Medical Association (JAMA)
http://jama.ama-assn.org/. Users can search archives and view full-text articles (including dozens on bird flu).

The Journal of Infectious Diseases
http://www.journals.uchicago.edu/JID/home.html. The premier publication in the western hemisphere for original research on the pathogenesis, diagnosis, and treatment of infectious diseases; on the microbes that cause them; and on disorders of host immune mechanisms. Articles in *JID* include research results from microbiology, immunology, epidemiology, and related disciplines.

Nature
http://www.nature.com/nature/focus/birdflu/index.html

The New England Journal of Medicine
http://content.nejm.org/cgi/content/full/353/13/1374. September 29, 2005 "Avian Influenza A (H5N1) Infection in Humans" (can search for other related articles).

New Scientist (UK magazine)
http://www.newscientist.com/channel/health/bird-flu. Compilation of original bird flu news.

Science
http://www.sciencemag.org. Founded in 1880 by inventor Thomas Edison, *Science* has grown to become the world's leading outlet for scientific news, commentary, and cutting-edge research, with the largest paid circulation of any peer-reviewed general-science journal. The journal is truly international in scope; some 35 to 40 percent of the corresponding authors of its papers are based outside the United States.

Scientific American
http://www.sciam.com/. Journal focusing on developments in science and technology. Need subscription to access all online content.

Journal of Virology
http://jvi.asm.org. (Only available to subscribers.)

Blogs

Avian Flu
What we need to know: http://avianflu.typepad.com/. News articles and commentary updated daily. Contains dozens of links to other sites and Asian news sources.

Bird Flu Watch
http://tahilla.typepad.com/birdflu/. Commentary-free list of news articles from around the world.

Flu Wiki
http://www.fluwikie.com/index.php?n=Main.HomePage. A variety of resources on avian influenza, from FAQ to aid opportunities to audio/video presentations and interviews with experts.

H5N1—News and Resources about Avian Flu
http://crofsblogs.typepad.com/h5n1/. Great blog, includes dozens of international links to other blogs, news sources, and health agencies, and details on bird flu books.

Wikipedia—Avian Influenza
http://en.wikipedia.org/wiki/Bird_flu. From Wiki, the Internet "encyclopedia." Basic information and dozens of good links.

Advocacy Groups

The Center for Consumer Freedom
http://www.consumerfreedom.com/. A nonprofit coalition of restaurants, food companies, and consumers working together to promote personal responsibility and protect consumer choices. Links to bird-flu related commentary and news, including article citing poll in which 47 percent of Americans said they believe they can acquire the bird flu by eating poultry.

Trust for America's Health (TFAH)
http://healthyamericans.org. TFAH is a nonprofit, nonpartisan organization dedicated to saving lives by protecting the health of every community and working to make disease prevention a national priority.

Miscellaneous

Nemours Foundation
http://kidshealth.org/teen/infections/colds_and_flu/bird_flu.html. Bird flu fact sheet specifically for teenagers.

The Flu Clinic Discussion Forum
http://www.curevents.com/vb/forumdisplay.php?f=40. Forum with more than 10,000 posts from people interested in discussing the flu (primarily bird flu).

Individualist: Bird Flu
http://health.groups.yahoo.com/group/individualist/. Yahoo! Groups discussion forum on bird flu.